Dear
Enjoy the
Good Info

Love

DAD

Hardwired for Love

Nurturing yourself to vibrant health

ALSO BY

HELENE B. LEONETTI, M.D.

From Little Lion & the Yggdrassill:
Bridging The Gap: 21st Century Healing for Women
(1998)

From Bridger House Publishers:
Menopause A Spiritual Renaissance (2002)

From Insight Publishing:
A Healthier You: Fabulous Ideas to Help You
Live a Healthier Life (2005)

From Little Seed Publishing:
Living in Clarity
(From the Wake Up...Live The Life You Love Series)
(2008)

From Morgan James:
Inspiring Hope: Stories of Hopeful
Living for More Success (2009)

Hardwired for Love

Nurturing yourself to vibrant health

HELENE B. LEONETTI, M.D.

Founder of the Self-Esteem Gene™

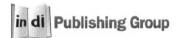 Publishing Group

Phoenix, Arizona

Hardwired for Love

Nurturing yourself to vibrant health

www.HardwiredForLove.com

Copyright © 2009 by Helene B. Leonetti, M.D.

All rights reserved.

INDI Publishing Group, www.INDIPublishingGroup.com.

Although the author and publisher have made every effort to ensure the accuracy and completeness of information contained in this book, we assume no responsibility for errors, inaccuracies, missions or any inconsistency herein. Any slights of people, places, or organizations are unintentional.

Printed and bound in the United State of America.

First printing 2009

Published by INDI Publishing Group in association with the author, Helene B. Leonetti, M.D.

Interior design by Julia Baumann
Cover design by Graham Van Dixhorn and Kathi Dunn

ISBN 13: 978-0-9789247-3-7 (13)

ISBN 10: 0-9789247-3-8 (10)

Library of Congress Control Number: 2009935095

ATTENTION CORPORATIONS, UNIVERSITIES, COLLEGES, AND PROFESSIONAL ORGANIZATIONS: Quantity discounts are available on bulk purchases of this book for educational, gift purposes, or as premiums for increasing magazine subscriptions or renewals. Special books or book excepts can also be created to fit specific needs.

For information, please contact INDI Publishing Group:
www.INDIPublishingGroup.com.

To Ida Louise DeLuca Leonetti

My precious mother, who,
unlike her daughter
did not ever come to know

> her enough-ness
> or her divinity.

May she reign over the angel realms,
teaching them cooking,

> baking, and
> crafts,

through which every atom
she wove her love.

Contents

Foreword

When I first met Dr. Helene Leonetti some years ago in Pennsylvania, I was immediately impressed by a sense of what might be called mutual harmonies-we seemed to be on the same wavelength-as if we'd been friends for years. For someone so petite, she radiated a sense of forthrightness that reminded me of that rare quality called true grit. Over time, I came to realize that her intellectual powers are amazingly well integrated with her heart and soul. She is that rare person who has arrived at a plane of development in which integrity, honesty and love permeates all phases of her life. This wonderful little book is the culmination of her personal character fulfillment. Using candid descriptions of her own pivotal life experiences, she communicates a path of life choices that turns obstacles into opportunities, doubts into convictions, anxieties into confidence, bad health practices into healing forces, and fear into love. Underlying all of this is her faith that, for true health and happiness, one must first love and honor one's own self and all others, since God loves us all despite our shortcomings. We must take charge in honoring that love by adopting healthy life choices: we have the power to be the best that we can be, regardless of circumstances. Her life and her health wisdom provide good direction for all of us to follow. Enjoy the book!

John R. Lee, M.D.

Acknowledgements

Thalia, my Greek soul sister who helped open my soul to true love;

Helen Paulus, my sage sister-in-heart who never let me sell out to my not-enoughness;

Tahya, elegant new friend and business associate who blends my teaching with her magnificent dance to teach self esteem;

Rose Moyer, my wonderful friend, born with the veil, who loves, and loves, and loves some more;

My son, Basil Leonetti, a major star in my firmament, who taught me mother love;

Deepak Chopra, who gave me courage to come out of the closet as a spiritualist;

Diane Cummings, my editor, whose wisdom and courage to know the essence of me created a masterful work in progress;

And on top, beloved Jakob: thank you for waiting.

Introduction

I went to college, medical school, and served a residency for twelve years, and no one ever taught me how to keep my patients healthy.

As a nurse in training in the sixties I was taught that doctors are gods and that we are to believe in their absolute authority. Through those years and the ones that followed when I was studying to become a doctor, I came to realize how disempowering that attitude was. It did not give room for the individual to rely on his/her own knowledge, understanding and experience.

There is a lot right within the conventional medical community, yet there is a lot wrong too. One has only to look at how we doctors are trained, and that should be enough to raise eyebrows about our ultimate wisdom. During our medical training and ensuing intern and resident years, we are deprived of the sleep required to adequately carry out our complex duties. And what does the medical establishment do about it? Nothing. It takes the legislature to pass a law requiring residents not to work over a certain number of hours without rest, so that the patients they serve will be protected from our mishaps, misdiagnoses and mistreatments.

We are taught nothing about healthy foods. Instead, we subsist on empty nutrition, high caffeine and sugar diets that ultimately burn out our adrenal glands and lower our immune states. We go from those long hours in the trenches home to study and then to bed, so that we rarely exercise, relax, have fun or smell the roses. Then we are expected to be sensitive, loving and caring with our patients when we have taken no time at all to nurture ourselves. *Who* has all the wisdom?

Our old conditioning tells us that viruses and bacteria cause disease and that most illnesses are hereditary, so that our ability to stay healthy is not within our grasp. Well, folks, it is time to get rid of that old, worn-out thinking, because we can free ourselves to recreate our destinies with new, healthy, and joyful beliefs.

Some years back, I saw the Light. My journey into true healing came serendipitously when I discovered the physician and author, Deepak Chopra's, message: that each and every cell in our bodies is connected, that all of our cells are thinking cells, and further, that every word and every thought and every action produces a *chemical* or *biophysical* reaction within our bodies. It is pretty awesome, isn't it, to think about what this means: *we control our own destinies.*

I have a recurrent dream in which our powerful HMOs will one day give referrals *first* to the herbalist, the chiropractor, the naturopath, the homoeopathist, the massage therapist and the acupuncturist before prescribing pills or sending patients to surgery. I daresay more of us conventionalists would rapidly learn the tenets of natural healing.

I regularly go to a chiropractor and acupuncturist and receive the blessed healing touch of a therapeutic massage therapist. Through them I have experienced major improvement from a chronic low back ailment. In the past I had also counseled with a psychotherapist who has helped me get in touch with my inner world. Now, I am in a perfect place of knowing, at a deep level, how vital these healing modalities are and how marvelously they interface with what I do as a gynecologist.

I have looked at the exciting role that I play in my patients' lives, and I realize that it in no way resembles the conventional doctor-patient relationship. Many years ago as a budding nursing student, I was admonished never to address patients by their first names, and to respectfully stand by their bedside, not to sit, and "contaminate" the bed linen. Well, thank God, I never resonated to such prattling, because I have come to learn that it is the intimacy with which we share our stories that brings about healing. I have learned that healing, true healing, takes place not only on the physical level but also more importantly, on our emotional bodies and deep within the soul.

Recently, I began a new lecture and class: "The Self Esteem Gene: Tapping into your Soul's Wisdom and Harnessing Your Personal Power." After discussing my years of dysfunctional relationships, then revealing how grace facilitated my healing, we sit in a circle with a talking stick and share our powerful stories. These sessions are a light that shines like a beacon, nurturing us, healing us, and reminding us that we are indeed magnificent.

Now that I know beyond a doubt the power of the body-mind-spirit connection, I can teach my wonderful patients how to empower themselves to find the physician within themselves. We are indeed spiritual beings learning to be human, and the realization of our soul potential is the most exciting part of this magnificent journey.

I want you along as we embark on a most wonderful and exciting journey into self-healing. The secret to health is self-love and empowerment, achieved when knowledge is attained of the multiple and diverse ways to arrive at and maintain a healthy mind, body, and spirit, not one of which can work without the others.

Part I

The
Hormone
Connection

CHAPTER 1

Confessions of a Goddess

Let me tell you a story about someone I know. She was a pretty thing: born an only child to two adoring parents. Mom sewed her clothes from the time she was a wee one. She was voted best dressed in high school and May queen in eighth grade. For as long as she could remember, she was boy crazy. At age eleven, she walked home from school, adoring the boy we shall call Darin who walked on the other side of the street. Darin never spoke to her, never shared a story with her, but she concocted a fantasy that brought them together nonetheless.

The girl's love life seemed to progress in high school. Freddie, the basketball hero, chose her for his girlfriend. But he wasn't very reliable and he seemed very arrogant. He might, or might not, show up for their dates together. The girl would sit in her bedroom, peering out the Venetian blinds, most often in vain, for his hotrod. On the occasions he did show, no apologies, no explanations. Freddie liked her mother's chocolate chip cookies, maybe more than he liked her. But our girl never complained nor did she ask for more in this lopsided relationship. Was she lucky that this fellow, coveted by so many other girls, had chosen her? She must, after all, be someone special.

As high school drew to an end with graduation looming, the girl sought out her guidance counselor querying her about the future. What she could be, as she entered this time when careers were being entertained? The answer she received was stark and terse: you are a woman; you can be a nurse or a teacher.

Being an obedient teen, our girl chose nursing because she felt drawn to the nurturing aspects of caring for the sick. So a registered nurse she became. She looked dashing in her nursing uniforms, with their charming caps and black velvet ribbons certifying her status.

As she grew, so did her beauty. She was wined and dined by many interns and residents. In each relationship—and they followed one after another in swift succession—she gave herself completely, vowing eternal love and commitment. But for all of her devotion, she was regularly dumped. These doctors, after all, were in training. They had hard years ahead with debt piling up. They were looking for distraction, not eternal love.

Around the age of twenty-six, while working in Montefiore Hospital in the Bronx, our girl was reminded by her Italian family that single professional women wound up old maids, and without marriage to a man with a future, her own future would be dire. Obedient girl that she was, she allowed herself to be fixed up with the brother of her cousin's workmate. Her marriage was expected and "arranged" accordingly.

It was a storybook wedding, followed by a magnificent honeymoon in Curacao. Then reality set in and she wasn't ready for it.

When she fell in love with a towering, intellectual professor at her hospital, her guilt surfaced and the affair was revealed. At home, the physical abuse, which had shown itself subtly during their engagement, exploded into terror-filled days and nights and worsened with the erratic nature of the beatings. Our girl was never sure when the seemingly placid surface would be eroded by uncontrollable anger. She stayed, she was a bad woman, she deserved the beatings.

For a brief time in this eleven-year marriage there was peace, a kind of truce. She was living in Mississippi. She conceived and birthed her beloved son while her husband attended law school. He completed three years. Straight As. All was well. And then a political incursion erupted, and he was expelled, persona non grata, with no hopes of securing entry into another school.

Moving back in defeat to New Jersey, the beatings escalated. Her son was now three years of age and witnessing the abuse. One day, while tending to bacon sizzling on the stovetop, a sobbing overwhelmed her, and tears splashed down, crackling into the bacon drippings. She realized that she did not like what she had become as a result of this marriage.

Deciding finally to leave, she was faced with pleadings to stay, but her need to go to medical school was pressing. Believing that her son would be better off with his father as she traveled to foreign shores, she was devastated years later to find that her husband's anger had settled onto his son, who became the focus of his rage.

Fast forward, fast forward: Medical school was complete, and a magnificent Brit entered her life during residency. Her marriage to this adoring man seemed to be the answer to her prayers: she finally felt loved to the extent she craved, and she plotted to leave medicine so that she could spend all her time with him. Alas, the Universe has a wicked sense of humor, for as they made love one night a short time into their marriage, he suffered a massive heart attack and died in her arms.

Stuffing her grief, our girl threw herself into her residency, delivering babies, operating on women with ruptured ectopic pregnancies. Her only solace.

Then enter husband number three. He wooed her, promising a

magnificent and wonderful life. She married him with great trepidation because she sensed his controlling ways. But she already had succumbed, and then life catapulted into a black abyss of fear and despair, which one was more consuming, she could not say.

Plotting one's death with such laser-sharp precision cannot even be given words. But her misery so complete, her joy so entirely lacking, and her consuming need for reprieve from pain muted all that might be pleasurable. She could no longer plan for the future, revel in the song of a bird, be dazzled by the beauty of a rose, or share in the hopes and dreams of her son. Her suicide attempt was thwarted, though, and she awoke in a hospital bed enraged to be viewing a bright sunshiny day and a nurse peering down at her with contempt.

Still asleep, she engaged her fourth husband, this time a spiritualist who taught meditation and engaged her and assisted her in writing her teachings and memoirs. This ten-year odyssey crumbled as she recognized that *she* was the wind beneath *his* wings, and not the other way around, as he had told her and she had once thought.

In a fascinating parallel to those many years ago, she found herself cooking bacon, again, weeping uncontrollably, her tears again falling into the sizzling pan.

"What does bringing home the bacon mean to you?" asked one of her best friends, Helen Paulus.

Hmm... she finally acknowledged that she had financially supported husbands in two of her marriages, stuffing the anger and despair it caused. Finally she left this fourth husband, and at least, so she thought, was at the top of her game. She was a published author, Reiki master, researcher, respected holistic gynecologist. She had it all.

But wait a minute. Did she still have lessons to learn?

The man she had loved throughout medical school and in

between all these marriages came strongly into her mind. She remembered with shame that for each of her last three marriages, she had dumped him. It had been almost sixteen years since she had seen or spoken to him, but now she felt an inexplicable urge to reconnect. She knew she could not rest until she moved on her feeling. Her reunion with this man would be her final waterloo and would catapult her toward a showdown with herself.

Despite living sixty-six years on this planet, I can truly say that only in the past two of those years I have learned to love myself unconditionally. What are you talking about, you ask? You, who accomplished great things against obstacles most would have thought too daunting to attempt. Yes, I respond, I know. I went to medical school in Mexico near the age of forty; I entered a competitive surgical subspecialty at forty-five when most are winding down into a kinder, gentler practice. And I studied herbalism, and bio-identical hormones, and spirituality, incorporating them into use with my patients, despite my being called "quack" by many of my colleagues.

During a profound depression, my ego finally gave way, and that would change the way I viewed myself and the world I inhabited. Menopause was the impetus that let me die to my old self and rebirth the new me that has come full circle into self-respect, and self-love.

Beloveds, I am here today, despite forty years of drama, to let you know that healing, that perfect health, continues to be our birthright. We are on a journey to this healing. I want my story to give you the courage to begin yours.

CHAPTER 2

Menopause:
A Spiritual Renaissance

Each person carries his own doctor inside.
Patients come to us not knowing that truth.
We are at our best when we give the doctor
who resides within each patient
a chance to go to work.
—Albert Schweitzer

Do you know of the marvelous work by Clarissa Pinkola Estes called
Women Who Run With the Wolves? *You know now that if you read*
the Bluebeard story you will get a picture of me. I was a chief resident
when I met my soon-to-be third husband, the Robert Redford look-alike
with a CV from here to Mars, who wined, dined and pursued me
relentlessly until I gave up and married him, knowing that it was to be
a deadly mismatch. I had lost my identity, and all my joy and
spontaneity, which had so attracted me to him, slid into oblivion, as I
catapulted deeper and deeper into the abyss of depression. Couple this
with a profound sense of my own inferiority at becoming the great
white physician after having been the obedient nurse—I was once
made to stand when a physician entered the room, add a pathetic total

absence of self-esteem, and include shouldering the anger and resentment of a sixteen-year-old son desperate to be accepted by a new stepfather who had no regard for children, and I was, to say the least, vulnerable. What tossed me over the edge was a condition that I would subsequently devote much of my professional life to exploring— Menopause.

My periods were becoming scant and irregular, and finally, feeling rotten from anti-depressant medications, I started to take hormone replacement therapy. I wish I could report that these hormones were making me feel better; perhaps the hot flashes improved, but my overall sense of despair did not. Using my body and my soul as a laboratory lesson, I launched into studying everything I could about menopause and vowed to be the best teacher I could be.

The literature in the industrialized world is replete with allusions to the multiple emotional upheavals associated with menopause and hormone imbalance. Needless to say, this information is fueled by the medical-pharmaceutical industrial complex, which, by their very connection with pathology, take a meaningful transition in a woman's life and transform it into a nightmare of parchment paper-like vaginas, bones that crack and break, and hearts doomed to suffer fatal attacks.

I was never taught in medical school that menopause is a natural life transition, one that signals entry into a magnificent state of wisdom and power. But I have learned on my own that it is.

One of the many areas where we are stuck is in old thinking about menopause. We are led to believe that when we reach our late forties or early fifties beauty fades, our sexual desirability wanes, and we risk multiple chronic illnesses. Nothing could be farther from the truth. Our loving Creator provided us women with this special time in life to recognize the true essence of our being. It is no coincidence, though, that as menopause approaches we do experience some dramatic bodily changes: hot flashes and night sweats, sexual dysfunction, hair loss or unwanted hair growth, constipation, weight gain, bleeding, depression and brain fog. God in His/Her incredible wisdom provided these gifts in order to nudge us into seeking help for our own needs. After all, think just how long we have been nurturing everyone else's needs instead of our own.

I began some years ago giving monthly lectures called *The Good News about Menopause,* a seeming oxymoron for many women. I wanted all women to understand that menopause is not the beginning of the end, but indeed is a spiritual renaissance, the beginning of the *best* time in life. Many women need to be helped through to this attitude, and it is my mission to remind them, and their significant others, of that fact. For seven years, in a monthly healing circle, known as *A Menopausal Enrichment Circle for Women,* a gathering co-facilitated by a psychotherapist, we set the stage for a safe and sacred space where women could share their dreams, fears, and often-traumatic stories of their journey toward wholeness.

I have sought not to "medicalize" the subject of menopause, where menopausal women become victims of the powerful medical-pharmaceutical complex. Rather, my approach is that menopause is a natural state, not a medical condition, and that it can, indeed must, be considered from a view of wholeness, connecting together the body, mind and spirit. In fact, what I ultimately recognized was that until you put your body, mind and spirit in order, all the pharmaceuticals in creation will not help. And further, promoting dependence on a chemical existence, which has been the basis of our medical philosophy over these last fifty years, continues to keep patients victims and the great white father physicians our saviors. (Our Asian sisters and those in third world nations snicker at our obsession with synthetic pharmaceuticals that we think will save our lives.)

So come along with me, my sisters, and see how we can make menopause a magnificent journey.

Take Home Pearls

✧ Menopause is not a disease: This change of season signals a time of great power when we complete our fertile years and move into our wise-woman years.

✧ Symptoms of flashes, insomnia, brain fog, anxiety are our friends, come to remind us of our imbalance

✧ Self love, taking our needs *first*, is key!

CHAPTER 3

Estrogen Myths – Progesterone Magic

Seek not to find out who you are,
seek to determine who you want to be.
—Neale Donald Walsch

As a new graduate nurse working in Montefiore Hospital in the Bronx, I was particularly idealistic and fiercely protective of my patients. One day as I cared for Mr. Artusi, a delightful man in his mid-thirties, an entourage of physicians and those-to-be descended into his room like Attila and his forces—all power and business. There, preceding the pack was Dr. Ackerman, chief of Orthopedics. He was followed by his chief resident, his junior residents, his interns, the medical students, and lastly, the pre-medical observer, a being swooning over the hallowed profession of medicine and praying for admission to the hallowed halls among these god-like beings.

Mr. Artusi had a dangerous infection of his hipbone, called osteomyelitis, and although he was on massive doses of long-term antibiotics, the specialists feared he was not healing. As they marched in, they began their medical blathering without even acknowledging this patient's presence, not even saying hello. The chief resident presented his case to the great Dr. Ackerman, as if the patient were a cadaver. The discourse proceeded through the history of the present illness, past medical history, family's medical history, social history, the proposed treatment, and finally the prognosis. The patient looked on terrified, as if he was hovering over his own funeral. Finally, the troops turned and marched out, ready to descend on yet another pathology specimen.

I was so incensed that my Italian temper, which rarely surfaced, now rose full-force, and I raced down the hall after God ... oops ... I mean Dr. Ackerman. He was a tall man and I, barely over five-feet, had to strain up on tippy toes to look him in the eye.

"You know, you didn't even have the common decency to say hello to this patient or ask him how he felt," I admonished. "What kind of a doctor are you?"

Dr. Ackerman just stared at me, perplexed. He simply didn't get it.

I was amazed and disgusted, yet grateful for this experience because it marked a turning point for me. You see, doctors are not—or at least they haven't until recently—been taught the least measure of civility. They have not known to place the sensitivities and emotional well being of a patient on an equal footing with his physical health.

And I now understand so well that healing needs to be invited by several modalities: definitely a look at the patient's history and prognosis. But incorporated into treatment must come emphasis on many other elements including nutrition.

Since my entry into the caring professions as a nurse in 1961, I have been counseled about the benefits of estrogen replacement therapy (ERT) for the menopause. Estrogen is touted in magazines, medical journals and on TV talk shows. We medical doctors are taught that without estrogen women will sustain life-threatening fractures, die in great numbers of cardiovascular disease, become old and lose their zest for life.

This view is largely the responsibility of a doctor named Robert Wilson, who wrote a book called *Forever Feminine,* in which he described women who did not replace their falling estrogen stores in menopause as virtual shadows of their former selves, destined to become dried up, sexless hags with no one willing to love them. A woman with flagging self-esteem didn't have to read much of that nonsense before she ran to her physician for some of the magic potion. And indeed, during the sixties and seventies, doctors were prescribing for women large and pervasive doses of estrogen.

We women were given a bum steer for all of those years, and sadly, we bought into it. How fascinating that in spite of the fact that menopause is a universal event, only in our modernized western societies, particularly America, do we pressure women into a mindset that espouses menopause as veering into a decrepit state which only a pill can fix. And sadly, I must remind you, we learn this from the seminars and journals and conferences that are sponsored and subsidized by the mammoth pharmaceutical industry.

A BIG BLUNDER

During the time from the late 1950s through the seventies, while women were given these large estrogen doses, problems developed. It was discovered that about 4 percent of the women taking estrogen developed uterine cancer. Because of that discovery, it was seen that another substance had to be added to protect the uterine lining. That substance, developed by the drug companies was a synthetic progesterone, called progestin (branded Provera). But it had many nasty side effects, and women began refusing to have anything to do with hormone replacement therapy of any kind. Women who suffered erratic bleeding during menopause finally invariably submitted to hysterectomies.

Today we know more, but we're still behind the times. Synthetic estrogen and synthetic progesterone are still around, and they're still creating a fair amount of havoc. Although only 15 percent of American women use estrogen because they fear the increased risk of breast cancer, most doctors persisted in encouraging its application. Even more confounding is the fact that most women experiencing menopausal symptoms, for which estrogen is prescribed, are actually estrogen dominant: their bodies have too much estrogen!

A LITTLE BACKGROUND

To explain: as we progress through our thirties into our forties, many of our menstrual cycles are an-ovulatory; that is, they produce no eggs. These an-ovulatory cycles can occur regularly or they can be erratic and heavy, filled with multiple clots and severe cramping. These cycles can also be accompanied by an array of disturbing symptoms that send women streaming to doctors' offices: water retention and edema, breast swelling, fibrocystic breasts, mood swings, depression, loss of libido, pelvic pain (a sign of possible uterine fibroid tumors), sugar cravings, and weight gain, noticeably at the hips and thighs. The accepted prescription for relief of these symptoms is the synthetic hormone, estrogen. *But did you know that all of these symptoms could be indications of too much estrogen?* So, there is a good chance that when estrogen is being prescribed to *alleviate* these symptoms, it is actually acting to *elevate* them. And the patient's distress becomes *more pronounced.*

Now, it is important to understand that during menopause

women do in fact lose some estrogen stores, but not all, usually between 40 and 60 percent. Our sumptuous sisters with extra body fat lose less, as estrogen hangs out in our fat cells.

During a woman's fertile years, she produces three primary hormones: estrogen, progesterone and testosterone. These three work hand-in-hand, synergistically, during these reproductive years, and they maintain a healthy balance.

But during the an-ovulatory cycles, where no eggs are produced, no progesterone is produced either. And estrogen builds relative to the absence of progesterone. So, during the many years between our mid thirties all the way into our late fifties, with erratic ovulation, there is little to no proges-terone to balance estrogen; hence, unpleasant symptoms develop.

Here's my take: no woman will ever be totally deficient in estrogen, because even if her uterus and ovaries are removed, estrogen will still be made through a conversion process in the adrenal glands. Conversely, most women stop making progesterone earlier than we ever dreamed.

GETTING IT WRONG

When in the sixties, doctors got that progesterone was needed to balance estrogen and the synthetic progesterone (progestin) was developed and widely prescribed for menopausal women, there came with it one big problem. Progestins don't work. Synthetic progesterone can make one and only one claim to fame: it controls the stimulatory effects of estrogen on the uterine lining and prevents the risk of cancer. But at a steep price: it *inhibits* the body's utilization of the *natural hormone, progesterone*; additionally, the synthetic progestins, such as the well-known Provera, can cause numerous conditions:

- breast tenderness with a milky discharge
- breakthrough bleeding and menstrual irregularities
- depression
- acne
- hair loss or hirsutism (hairy face, body)
- headaches
- PMS
- high blood pressure
- nervousness

What we have done in the past, and continue to do under the influence of our pharmaceutical industry, is to tout the benefits of synthetic progestins as if they were identical to *natural* progesterone. Friends, the synthetic progestin is no more like natural progesterone than apples are to bananas.

The case for natural progesterone is strong. Even the pharmaceutical industry is paying some attention to the press that natural progesterone is receiving and has introduced an oral medication, Prometrium. This certainly is better than the synthetic progestin, medroxyprogesterone (Provera) or aygestin, but because the oral progesterone gets rerouted through our intestinal tract, approximately 90 per cent of it is converted by the liver into metabolic byproducts that make us sleepy, dizzy, fatigued. Such side effects are, however, desired for insomniac women who get help by taking it before bedtime.

SO WHAT'S THE ANSWER?

There is another version of the hormone progesterone with many more compelling benefits and virtually no side effects: it is natural transdermal progesterone, a cream that is rubbed onto the skin.

Our skin is the most efficient organ for absorption. It boasts a significant attraction to the membrane of the red blood cell onto which it will piggyback as it absorbs.

I prescribe transdermal, or skin, progesterone cream, and the vast majority of my patients receive many benefits from it. The variety I prefer incorporates aloe and Vitamin E, which dry, craggy skin finds delicious and soaks up. And the other rewards are countless: natural transdermal progesterone can improve osteoporosis and cardiac function; it enhances thyroid function— you estrogen-only users may well suffer from hypo-thyroidism because estrogen locks up thyroid function, making it less efficient, while progesterone unlocks it, enhancing thyroid function; it protects against breast and uterine cancer and, because it has a cortisone-like action, it is an anti-inflammatory and helps with aches and pains. The bonus factor is that it revs up the sex drive.

I would like to caution you right now that not all natural progesterone creams are created equal. When buying, you should look for a product that contains between nine hundred and one thousand milligrams of progesterone for every two ounces of cream (¼ tsp = 20 mgs).

Do I ever prescribe ERT? Yes. Most women in peri-menopause who are still mensing but not producing progesterone will do beautifully on progesterone alone. For other women, lean and healthy women, who have gone one year without menstruating or who have had hysterectomies, and who may suffer symptoms—hot flashes, brain fog, decreased libido—for which progesterone alone will not be enough for relief, I prescribe estrogen. Usually I prescribe those made from natural soybean substances and delivered by patch, gel, spray or pill, though I am using less and less by mouth because of the initial metabolism through the liver which is already taxed with so many detoxifying jobs.

TESTOSTERONE FOR WOMEN?

Testosterone recently has been given attention as a hormone that needs to be replaced in menopausal women, particularly women who have lost their ovaries, because that is where, along with the adrenal glands, testosterone is produced. While women make much less testosterone than do men, still it is an important ingredient for maintaining well being and a lively libido. The pharmaceutical companies have come up with a replacement synthetic testosterone, but unfortunately it contains a methyl group, which has been shown to lower good cholesterol and to adversely affect the liver.

I prescribe a 2 percent natural testosterone cream and instruct my patients to use a lentil pea-size amount on the clitoris nightly. For women with vaginal dryness, weak bladders *and* decreased sexual desire, I order from a compound pharmacy a mixture of estriol—the safer estrogen made primarily when we are pregnant—and testosterone. I instruct patients to massage a garden-sized pea amount of cream into their vaginas nightly. This is usually 0.5 milligrams of each/1 gram.

I have particular appreciation for pharmacists, such as my friend, Pete Hueseman, who speak of the difference between synthetic and natural progesterone and who have additional training to make compounds of natural, bio-identical hormones. While I am certainly no fan of large doses of pharmaceutical estrogens, particularly those made from horse urine because of the cruelty suffered by our animal friends, I do prescribe plant estrogens— pharmaceutical and herbal—but *never* without natural progesterone.

You may wonder why many doctors seem to know nothing of

the natural hormone, progesterone, which is often all we need during the challenging years before, during and after menopause, and persist in prescribing synthetic progestins, which have many side effects, especially in light of the fact that the Women's Health Initiative (WHI) crashed three years prematurely in 2002 because of an unacceptably high amount of breast cancer, strokes, blood clots to the lungs, and heart attacks. WHI consisted of a set of clinical trials designed to test the effects of postmenopausal hormone therapy. What actually was solidified is that synthetic progesterone is more risky than estrogen.

I believe that much of the impasse surrounding physicians' refusal to get on board with the latest research results lies in the concept of what I term old wisdom: it is easier and safer to continue espousing common, conventional practice than to spend time and effort considering a diametrically opposing one, thus risking criticism, even ostracism, from one's colleagues.

There are some who support these "far out" theories, though. My pharmacist friend, Pete, writes in his article, *"A Pharmacist Explores Some Differences Between Natural Progesterone and Synthetic Progestin:"*

> We live in an era when more and more emphasis is being placed on the importance of natural substances. Natural food supplements and herbal formulations are in demand. Homeopathic physicians and caregivers are regaining popularity. Everyone seems to be asking, "What can we do to help the body repair itself in a more natural fashion?"
> Many women who take hormone replacement therapy are also asking the "natural vs. synthetic" question. Is natural always better? What is the difference between the natural progesterone and the synthetic progestin, medroxyprogesterone, also commonly prescribed as Provera?
> The most outstanding difference between the two is that medroxyprogesterone is an analog, a look-alike of

progesterone, not truly a progesterone at all, but rather a progestin. The chemical structure of medroxyprogesterone closely resembles the chemical structure of progesterone as it is produced naturally in the human body. But even a slight difference in the molecular configuration of a compound can produce a totally different response from its natural counterpart.

Progesterone is the oldest steroid hormone-some 500 million years old on the evolutionary scale. All vertebrates produce progesterone although it is only in higher vertebrates that this hormone is instrumental in the reproductive cycle. In lower vertebrates progesterone functions in relation to glucose metabolism, the development of intelligence, and bone formation.

The process of producing natural progesterone, which is made from yams and soybeans, was discovered by Russell Marker, a Pennsylvania State College chemistry professor. While experimenting with sapogenins, a group of plant steroids, in the jungles of Mexico in the 1930's, Marker realized that progesterone could be transformed by chemical process from a sapogenin, diosgenin, which is found naturally in yam.

Unlike medroxyprogesterone, natural progesterone is an exact chemical duplicate of the progesterone that is produced by the human body. Another immediate difference between medroxyprogesterone and natural progesterone is that the synthetic hormone can actually lower a patient's blood level of progesterone. Some women who take medroxyprogesterone to combat PMS or oppose estrogen in menopause, report headaches, mood swings, and fluid retention.

On the other hand, women who take natural progesterone often say that their mood swings diminish. Women who suffer from migraines as their main complaint with PMS also find that this situation may be corrected by natural progesterone. In its natural form, progesterone acts as a diuretic, which means that women who take these supplements may have to go to the bathroom more frequently, but they are spared the fluid retention and weight gain experienced by women on synthetic progestin.

Prescribed doses also differ in regard to natural and synthetic progesterone. Synthetic progestin is ten to one hundred times as potent as the natural progesterone. This appears to be a tremendous range, but the doses fall well within those limits ...

Synthetic progestins were developed with the advent of the birth control pill. The half-life of natural progesterone was very short and researchers were looking for an agent that would give a longer half-life and yet produce or mimic the effect of progesterone. Birth control pills contain, in most cases, a synthetic progestin and a synthetic estrogen. The very potent synthetic progestins prevent ovulation in a very low dose and, therefore, accomplish their function of birth control.

Conversely, natural progesterone has been used for many years in pregnancy, luteal phase defect, and postpartum depression. When a woman is pregnant, her progesterone levels are thirty to fifty times higher than normal. A nursing mother should not be concerned that taking natural progesterone for postpartum depression will affect the baby. After all, the baby has been exposed to tremendous levels of progesterone during pregnancy.

Significant difference exists between synthetic and natural progesterone. Natural progesterone duplicates the body's progesterone exactly, causes fewer side effects and can be more consistently utilized by the body. In the case of natural progesterone versus the synthetic progestins in hormone replacement, natural does appear to be better.

SAFE AND SANE

Obviously, you are asking, is natural progesterone safe? After all, my doctor doesn't know a thing about it; there is little on the subject in the medical journals, especially about the transdermal type, so why should I believe you?

Healthy skepticism is a wonderful virtue, a first step in your exciting journey to healing—never take anything at face value. But let me now help assuage your doubts.

The first breakthrough in acknowledging the benefits of natural progesterone shows up in an important study called PEPI.[1]

Five different arms of hormone replacement therapy were used to evaluate how hormones protect the cardiovascular system. Four of the study arms used synthetic progestin and/or estrogen. The fifth arm used estrogen along with natural progesterone. The results surprised everyone, because the "fifth arm" women who used natural progesterone showed an improved lipid profile: good cholesterol (HDL) numbers went up; bad cholesterol figures (LDL) went down. In addition, no excessive bleeding occurred, and the uterine lining was equally protected against an overgrowth of estrogen dominant tissue. Use of the synthetic progesterone (medroxyprogesterone), showed that the positive effects of estrogen on HDLs, or high-density lipoproteins, were muted, or lessened. In fact, in many instances LDLs, or low-density lipoproteins, actually rose.

A magnificent study performed at the Primate Center in Oregon further demonstrates this.[2] In this study, menopausal rhesus monkeys were divided into two groups: one group was put on the synthetic progesterone, Provera, while the other group was given natural progesterone. Then both groups of monkeys were dosed with a drug known to cause arteries to squeeze close. In the case of the monkeys given natural progesterone, the arteries stayed open. The monkeys with Provera suffered blocked arteries.

I call synthetic progesterone the look-alike drug that women love to hate, as it promotes severe PMS symptoms—anxiety, headaches and bloating, conditions most often absent with natural

[1] Post-Menopausal Estrogen/Progestin Interventions Trial (PEPI). The Writing Group for the PEPI Trial. *JAMA* (1995) 273 (3): 199-208.

[2] R. D. Minshall, et al. "Ovarian Steroid Protection Against Coronary Artery Hyperreactivity in Rhesus Monkeys," *Journal of Clinical Endocrinology and Metabolism* (1998) 83:2 649

progesterone.

Additional benefits make natural progesterone truly remarkable: it enhances thyroid function, acts as a natural anti-depressant, is a natural diuretic, protects against breast fibrocysts, breast cancer, and uterine cancer and is a stabilizer for metabolism of copper and zinc, whose balance is key to the brain's regulation of our mood swings and responses to stress. It also protects our bones against osteoporosis.

For skeptics concerned that transdermal progesterone is not systemically absorbed, my two published studies confirm that it is.[3,4]

---

[3] "Topical Progesterone Cream Has An Antiproliferative Effect on Estrogen-Stimulated Endometrium," FERTILITY AND STERILITY Vol 79, No 1, Jan 2003, pp 221-2

[4] "Transdermal Progesterone Cream as an Alternative Progestin in Hormone Therapy," ALTERNATIVE THERAPIES; Vol 11, No 6, Nov/Dec, 2005; pp36-8. Each was awarded third prize by the prestigious American College of OB-GYN, proving uterine protection equal to that of synthetic progestins when used with estrogen.

Take Home Pearls

✧ Natural plant estrogens are 'bioidentical' to what the body makes, whereas synthetic estrogens (horse urine) are not smart enough to trick the body into thinking they belong there. Horse urine is natural for horses, not humans.

✧ Estrogens are indicated for women who, despite natural progesterone, continue having symptoms of brain fog, anxiety, vaginal dryness; but they must be used cautiously in women with breast, uterine cancers.

✧ *All* women, regardless of whether they have had hysterectomy, with or without removal of ovaries, need natural progesterone to balance the estrogen they are given.

✧ Estriol is a very safe form of estrogen and needs to be provided by a compounding pharmacy.

✧ Natural progesterone used transdermally enhances thyroid function, protects our breast, heart, and bones, and assists with our sex drive.

✧ Testosterone in small amounts revs up our libido and used with estriol vaginally helps with dryness and bladder issues.

✧ Self love, taking our needs *first*, is key!

CHAPTER 4

Science and the Yam

Let the love you have be what you do.
—Rumi

During my nursing days in the sixties, the wards at Jersey City Medical Center were huge, housing some sixty patients. The female unit on one side of this medicinal environment, replete with peeling lead-based painted walls and without the cheery prints and potted plants of today, was lined with manual crank metal frame beds, with mattresses that to my fading memory were four to five inches thick. They were nothing like what we see today, those splendid beauty-rest varieties with endless position changing possibilities. While you can easily relate to the private and semi-private rooms of contemporary day hospitals, when I say wards, I mean just that--fourteen or so sparse beds separated only by muslin curtains. The travails, painful moans, and fearful tears were shared communally.

Katie was one of my favorite patients. She was all of four feet eight inches tall, eighty-eight pounds, and stooped with the ravages of osteoporosis. She was gorgeous, nonetheless, all seventy-eight years of her: she possessed a thick white mane, long and lustrous, which I often combed and braided, using for ribbons the gauze that served in hospitals as wash cloths. Katie's soul shone through her large crystal-clear blue eyes.

"Ah, Girl," she would say, (however many times I told her my name, she preferred calling me girl), "I am so scared: my cat and my television are alone in my apartment and I am afraid my cat will starve and the vandals will steal my TV. What am I to do?"

Katie lived in a rent-controlled apartment in a once opulent area since gone shabby by the influx of people not loving themselves and their environment enough to treat their neighborhoods with respect.

Well, I did what any loving nurse would do: one day after my seven to three shift ended, I drove over to Katie's apartment and found the landlord, who generously took Katie's cat and TV set into his own apartment until she was discharged.

I was happy to help Katie, even though she had not directly asked me to. Then I wondered, why is it so difficult to ask for help? The Bible says ask and it shall be given. I think that too often we are afraid to ask because we feel so unworthy that we can't believe anyone else would be interested in coming to our aid.

What we must remember always is that we are mirror images of each other: when we feel lower than low about ourselves, so also do others view us. I think about Katie when I feel a need to empower myself with self-love.

FOUR STUDIES

Plenty of evidentiary research exists to support the claims about natural progesterone, the miraculous hormone drawn from the humble yam.

The first study I share comes from Upsala, Sweden.[5] The study followed a group of 128 postmenopausal women with cancer of their uterine lining. Each patient underwent a procedure called D and C, where a portion of the uterine lining was scraped off, then analyzed to determine stages of disease. Also measured in the tumor mass and blood was S-phase fraction (SPF), which correlates the growth activity to the prognosis or prediction for the specific uterine cancer. Finally, the various hormones—progesterone, testosterone, and androstenedione, (a metabolic by-product of estrogen)—were measured. The latter two had no effect on the prognosis of the cancer. But, in the patients who maintained a certain level of progesterone concentration in their blood, there was a decrease in the tumor's proliferative, or spreading, ability: an indication of a possible healthier outcome.

For the next study, a brief crash course on the menstrual cycle will be helpful. In women with the average twenty-eight to thirty day cycle, the first fourteen days (approximately) are known as the proliferative or estrogenic phase; after this first phase comes mid-cycle, when we make an egg, or ovulate, and the uterine lining then converts to a predominantly secretory or progestational phase, dominated by progesterone production. If her consort, the sperm, does not meet the egg that bursts forth from the ovary, conception does not occur, and the uterine lining bleeds off, with day one beginning a new cycle. If we do not ovulate, we do not produce progesterone, period. Estrogen production, remember, never goes to zero, even when we have stopped our menses or if our ovaries have been removed. Estrogen continues to be made by our adrenal glands and is stored in our fat cells.

---

[5] K. Boman, M.D., et al. "The Influence of Progesterone and Androgens on the Growth of Endometrial Cancer," *Cancer* (1993) 71:3565-9.

Jerilynn C. Prior, M.D., of Vancouver, British Columbia, performed an exquisite and thorough study that furthers the case for the benefits of progesterone. It was called "Spinal Bone Loss and Ovulatory Disturbances."[6]

Originally, it was taught that only menopausal women and marathon runners of any age lose bone after estrogen begins to decrease. This very important study may have disproved this concept. Using three groups of pre-menopausal women, marathon runners, moderate exercisers, and women of regular activity between the ages of twenty-one and forty-two, Dr. Prior demonstrated that it is not a lack of estrogen that accounts for bone loss but rather the *lack of progesterone.* And she did so by revealing an-ovulatory cycles (remember: no ovulation, no progesterone) at least 29 percent of the time, in all three groups, regardless of their activity levels.

Very importantly, for those many women fearing the use of hormones because of the specter of breast cancer—good news! A skillfully done study from Taiwan and Paris[7] explored the effects of various hormones on cell growth in normal breast tissue. Forty women scheduled for removal of benign breast lumps were randomized into four groups and wore on the affected breast for two weeks prior to surgery a gel containing one of the following:

- Estrogen and progesterone
- Estrogen alone
- Progesterone alone

---

[6] J.C. Prior, M.D., et al. "Spinal Bone Loss and Ovulatory Disturbances," *New England Journal of Medicine* (1990) 323:1221-7.

[7] King-Jen Chang, M.D., et al. "Influences of Percutaneous Administration of Estradiol and Progesterone on Human Breast Epithelial Cell Cycle in Vivo," *Fertility and Sterility* (1995) 63:785-91.

- Placebo

After the breast lumps were removed, each was examined for cellular growth. As was expected, the estrogen lump showed an increase in the number of cycling cells. The mass under the influence of estrogen and progesterone revealed no change over the placebo group. But the most exciting finding was the progesterone group: there was an inhibition of the growth of cycling cells: this study strongly suggests that *progesterone acts to protect the breast.*

Lastly, molecular biologist and friend, Bent Formby, Ph.D., has carried out an excellent study worthy of the Nobel Prize.[8] Using human DNA breast cancer cell strains, he demonstrated that progesterone inhibits the growth of these cancer cells, while estrogen fuels this growth. He also found that progesterone fosters a phenomenon called *apoptosis*, or programmed cell death, which prevents conversion of normal cells into cancer cells. Additionally, he discovered that estrogen prevents apoptosis.

THE NATURAL WAY

I would not have stepped into this "natural healing" arena without the man I credit, most thankfully, for my enlightenment: the late John R. Lee, M.D. I knew him as an affable, formidable healer, a man far advanced in his thinking, who became my mentor as well as a blessed friend.

Dr. Lee began his journey as a family practitioner in Mill Valley, California. As he grew with his practice, his forty-year-old patients turned sixty, and with the progression of years came the recognition that their stooped shoulders were more than just world-weariness.

---

[8] Formby, Bent, Ph.D. et al. "Progesterone Inhibits Growth and Induces Apoptosis in Breast Cancer Cells: Inverse Effects on Bcl and p53," *Annals of Clinical and Laboratory Science*, Vol. 28, No.6: 2 and 53.

The well-known dowager's hump, named after the late British Queen Mum, was discovered not to have as much to do with old age so much as it did with compression fractures of the thoracic spine caused by osteoporosis.

As fate would have it, much that was to follow started in 1978 after he heard a lecture by Professor Ray Peat, Ph.D., of Blake College in Eugene, Oregon, about the various attributes of progesterone. It was from him that Dr. Lee learned about a skin cream, originally sold as a moisturizer, which contained among other ingredients, progesterone. He began recommending this cream to his aging women patients, and to his surprise, besides making them feel measurably better, their bone mineral density improved.

Dr. Lee noted that this gentle cream, delivered through the skin, has the distinct advantage of bypassing conjugation through the liver, which all oral medications have to do. Rubbing the cream into the skin directly delivers and circulates active progesterone into the system.

And remember, how much less of the cream we have to use. When taken orally, the traditional dose is one hundred to two hundred milligrams. When applied to the skin, transdermally, we only require twenty to forty milligrams (one-quarter to one-half teaspoon), five to ten times less!

My friend, David Zava, Ph.D., a biochemist and breast cancer researcher, has quantified these dosages. He analyzes the amounts of progesterone (as well as the steroid hormones: estrogen, testosterone, cortisol and DHEA), in saliva fluid that accurately reflects the active portion of progesterone in the body. Through this method, he has been able to assure the accuracy of the progesterone doses.

DOUBTING DOCTORS

The physicians who doubt the veracity of natural transdermal progesterone come to their conclusions through measurements of progesterone in blood serum. But, truly, looking for progesterone in this way is somewhat like looking outside for the car keys you dropped in the house. Transdermal progesterone is lipophilic, or lipid loving; it latches onto the fatty membrane of the red blood cells, hitching a ride in the blood, so to speak. Well, when conventional levels of progesterone are measured in the blood serum, the count is inaccurate because we have effectively spun down the blood, throwing the red blood cells away and using instead the straw-colored fluid to measure levels. But our detractors gleefully plot to discredit the skin cream by condescendingly pointing out that transdermal progesterone is not absorbed. "See," they taunt, "we told you it doesn't work: you cannot measure it in the blood!" The arrogance of ignorance keeps our blinders on to prevent us from seeing a new truth.

Dr. Lee entered one hundred women into a study[9] over three years and was astonished to see how much increase in bone density these women experienced after using transdermal progesterone cream. The average increase in bone density was close to 15 percent. The fascinating point is that he has disproved conventional medical teachings that insist that once bone is lost, it is gone forever.

Now, gentle readers, you can imagine the raucous behavior on the part of my conformist colleagues after reading this piece of news. Digging in their heels, they arrogantly reminded that the journal publishing this finding is truly insignificant, not prestigious, as is the *New England Journal of Medicine* or the *Journal of the American Medical Association,* or *Lancet.* Secondly, they were quick to point out that this was not a randomized, double-blinded, placebo-controlled

---

[9] *International Clinical Nutritional Review (*1990) 10:384-391.

study.

Very importantly (and sadly), no major pharmaceutical company sponsored the study, so it got little press, thus, little attention. Unfortunately, doctors learn how to use medications from the detail people who work for these megalithic pharmaceutical corporations. Natural transdermal progesterone gets little attention, because the pharmaceutical companies don't manufacture it.

The bottom line is that the miracle of natural progesterone is no longer hush-hush. For all the scientists out there, it is important to remember that progesterone *is* the master hormone. In the biochemical cascade, after cholesterol and pregnenolone, progesterone is the hormone from which testosterone, estrogen, and cortisol are made. In the human body, a small amount of estrogen and testosterone can be made from progesterone, but not the other way around.

THE WORK GOES ON

From the outset, I was excited about how natural progesterone was assisting so many women, and I felt motivated to carry on with what had gone before. In order to further mainstream credibility and give even more sober attention to the benefits of this "wonder cream," I constructed a randomized, double blind, placebo-controlled test. Along with my distinguished colleague, James Anasti, M.D., a brilliant reproductive endocrinologist who has done innumerable studies for the National Institutes of Health, I recruited 107 eligible women to participate in this most important study.

One remarkable finding was that after one year of research, we were able to show that 83 percent of the women using natural transdermal progesterone experienced relief from their hot flashes, while only 19 percent using the placebo cream did. These impressive statistics were published in the prestigious journal, *Obstetrics and Gynecology* in August 1999.

And this was just the beginning. We then studied sixty women, again in a randomized, double-blinded, placebo-controlled test, to find out whether the addition of natural progesterone for women using estrogen would protect the uterine lining against cancer. I'm pleased to say that our study was awarded third prize out of four hundred research projects submitted to the American College of Obstetrics and Gynecology, and our positive findings were presented at the College's May 2001 national convention.

Our third trial also received Third Prize for original research by ACOG and was published in 2005 Alternative Therapies. This definitive research followed twenty-six women, each of whom received a baseline endometrial biopsy and began a six-month course of Premarin and Provera. This was followed by another biopsy, a two week wash out period, then a six month course of Premarin (estrogen) and natural transdermal progesterone cream. Then a final biopsy of the uterine lining was done. The magnificent findings affirm that the natural progesterone cream gave as much protection to the uterine lining when used with estrogen as did the progestin. The pathologists were blinded to which women were on which arm of the study, so no prejudice could be rendered.

On a personal note, of course, I do not use Premarin in my practice: it is made of the horse urine obtained from a pregnant mare whose life is made hell with the cruel methods used to collect the urine. My decision to use Premarin in this study was a political one, since most conventional practitioners know only of Premarin and would have cast aside our findings if we had failed to use it.

As I stated in Chapter 3, I regularly prescribe estrogen, bio-identical estrogen, but I use the smallest doses I can, and always with the transdermal progesterone cream, which mutes the risk of cancer by the estrogen. I regularly use the safest form of estrogen, estriol, which has been used for decades in Europe, but which is not patented here in America. I recently learned that this is made here in America and sold in Europe, but our FDA has threatened to close down the companies that provide the hormone powder to our compounding pharmacies to make estriol. It could not be the giant pharmaceutical company, Wyeth, the makers of Premarin, influencing the FDA because of their great financial loss, could it be?

My fourth, and final, research trial, inspired by Dr. Lee, to whom I promised I would do the "little old lady study," is a two-year study, intending to recruit at least one hundred women seventy years of age and older to confirm—once and for all—with a placebo controlled, double blind study—that progesterone cream can prevent osteoporosis. My angel, John, is watching over us and will gleefully observe our success and finally be vindicated for his passionate life's work. To you, John, with love!

Who knew, God, that I would be the one to take on this divine mission!

Take Home Pearls

✧ Multiple studies, including mine, prove the safety of natural transdermal progesterone.

✧ Physiological doses of 20-40mg daily protect our thyroid, bones, breast, and hearts with *no* side effects.

✧ Self love, taking our needs *first*, is key!

CHAPTER 5

The Three Big Menopause Conundrums

There is nothing either good or bad, but thinking makes it so.
—Shakespeare

My medical school days in Mexico were filled with fun and joy; however, my playful nature would often land me in gut-wrenching trouble from which inevitably I would learn—the hard way—one of life's rigorous lessons.

I was living with a Mexican family, Alexandra, Refugio, and their daughter, Alex. Refugio was a judge, staid, respectable and somewhat aloof. His wife, Alexandra, on the other hand, was fun loving and adventurous, like me. She was twenty-seven to his forty-five years of age, which may have explained the contrast.

On my way home from classes each day, I would walk past a home adorned with a papaya tree on the front lawn, and each day I took note of the tree's prize: a mammoth, vibrantly colored, fully ripe papaya. It was the most enticing piece of fruit I had ever seen.

One evening after cena, the light evening meal consisting of scrambled eggs, tortillas, avocado slices, and limon—a cross between lemon and lime—I told Alexandra about the papaya, and we schemed to secure it for our own. Later that evening, with Refugio and their daughter safely tucked away in bed, we stole out, thieves in the night, with machete in tow, to descend on the unsuspecting victim.

While I kept watch, Alexandra pulled the knife from inside my sleeve and hacked off the coveted prize. We ran back home to enjoy the fruits of our shameful labor.

The next day, as I walked past that papaya tree, now missing its bounty, I saw a yellow ribbon tied about its trunk. Someone was mourning the loss. I couldn't have felt more bereft. I prayed to God to forgive my thievery, and I vowed never again to be a pirate.

POWER SURGES

The vasomotor flush, better known as the famous hot flash, is familiar to nearly 90 percent of all menopausal women. And we all know just exactly what a hot flash feels like. Without warning, the intense heat of a comet engulfs us, often starting at the head and neck and radiating occasionally to the chest. We turn beet red; we break out in intense perspiration, and that luscious silk blouse we wear so proudly and confidently sags like a limp, wet rag. At nighttime, we wake up drenched, feeling as if on fire. Then soon after our skin dries, we shiver with the cold. Off and back on go the covers all night long, and we awaken exhausted.

Though 75 percent of us experience spontaneous relief of these distractions after five years, the remaining 25 percent continue to suffer hot flashes, often throughout their lives.

The prevailing theory about the cause of the hot flash is that a part of the brain located near the pituitary, called the hypothalamus,

THE THREE BIG MENOPAUSE CONUNDRUMS

goes haywire because of falling levels of estrogen and progesterone, which had previously worked as an effective, well-oiled feedback mechanism to produce adequate amounts of these hormones. When the ovaries begin failing in their production of estrogen and progesterone, the substance from the hypothalamus, called gonadotrophic releasing *hormone* (GnRH), heightens its activity level and activates the vasomotor center, and flash! (no pun intended), we begin having flashes.

Traditionally we have been taught that it is estrogen deficiency that causes the flash, but the mechanism is much more complex than that. Natural progesterone, being the master hormone in the biochemical cascade, often relieves the debilitating symptoms. A partial explanation may be that since a small amount of estrogen and testosterone is manufactured in the body from progesterone, it alone is helpful. In fact, my first published research trial, if you remember from Chapter 4, demonstrated just that.

One very exciting fact is that if we begin using natural progesterone along with our estrogen, after a time we can cut the estrogen dose lower and lower and continue getting relief. This appears to occur because the progesterone increases the body's receptors for estrogen, and vice versa.

Since I started to use natural progesterone cream at age fifty-one, I first was able to cut my estrogen dose in half and have finally been able to wean off of it entirely. Now I use black cohosh and dong quai along with natural progesterone. My power surges have all but vanished, unless I am having a major league stress event. If I am, I deep breathe--slowly, and concentrate on ice cubes. Even so, my familiar friend comes to visit between seven and ten every night. However, I have chosen to look on this event differently. This rather imposing guest, my one great power surge, reminds me that my batteries need recharging. It is at this time, that I take a deep cleansing breath, express gratitude for all my blessings, and prepare to make way for another wonderful day.

At the North American Menopause Society meeting in Chicago in 1996, Suzanne Woodward, Ph.D., spoke about how women experiencing hot flashes, who are in a warm room two hours prior to sleep, will have many more hot flashes during the night than they would in a cool room. Cooling that room will suppress hot flashes.

When we delve into some alternative explanations for the hot flash, we begin to see again and again the body-mind-spirit connection. Carolyn Myss, a medical intuitive who originally worked with Norm Shealy, M.D., a neurologist and founding president of the American Holistic Medical Association, claims that hot flashes are related to blocked energy. She goes on to say that they are classic occurrences for non-orgasmic women who have experienced little sexual pleasure. Hmmm—food for thought.

In Vicki Noble's book, *Shakti Woman*, she reminds us of a well-documented fact: that high temperatures kill cancer cells and bacteria. She feels that hot flashes may be nature's way of killing off latent cancer cells so that we are protected as we move through our menopausal goddess years.

There are, obviously, many views on the whys and wherefores of the hot flash. It is perhaps time to view this circumstance not as the enemy but as simply an energy whose purpose is to move through us in order to move us to our own inner wisdom.

HAIR TODAY, GONE TOMORROW

When I was a young child, we lived in a railroad apartment on the third floor in Union City, New Jersey. Mom had worked as a beautician before having me, and my father was a magnificent Italian barber. I remember this as if it were yesterday, although up to the day they died—Mom at ninety-four, Dad at ninety-nine—they denied it, as they were kissing me good night, they told me that if I ever dared to touch my hair with any dye or bleach they would cut it off in the middle of the night! I probably dreamed that, but to this day, I have never added dye or bleach to my hair. Pretty heavy-duty programming, you might say!

Many of my patients come to see me with complaints that they have either too little hair or too much. A little bit like the Goldilocks story!

There are always some medical explanations, but like so many of the mysteries of life, many are only theories. It is easy to explain the menopausal changes in our facial hair: our hormones are going bonkers. Most of these changes are the result of an imbalance of estrogen, progesterone and testosterone, where all of a sudden we develop peach fuzz around the hairline, on our cheeks and chin, and accentuated sideburns. This can happen purely spontaneously or it can result from using testosterone cream too generously, a substance I promote once in a while to give the libido a gentle nudge.

The doctor in me will certainly check to see whether you have suddenly developed a male-pattern of hair growth on your chest, or abdomen or in the pubic area, because, along with a male-pattern baldness, this, in rare instances, could signal a tumor. But trust me, the vast numbers of hair issues are not life threatening. Just annoying and humiliating.

It is amazing to me how cultural mores determine how we see ourselves. In my father's homeland, Italy, women don't shave off the hair that sends American women in droves to electrolysis clinics and waxing boutiques. A thick mane of armpit or leg hair emerging from a European woman wearing a lavish ball gown is a perfectly acceptable sight.

My own neurosis centered on one large eyebrow. I had one thick eyebrow that ran across my forehead. So self-conscious was I that without my trusty tweezers, I would become hysterical. God forbid it should grow in all the way. But my friends would tease me and hide my tweezers until I could bear it no longer and panic set it. I learned at the tender age of twenty-four that tweezing hairs on your chin was not cool. Pluck one, and four arrive; pluck four and sixteen grow in to taunt you. Have the audacity to pluck sixteen, and you will have a full beard. I know: I did it. My mother confessor, Sally Gurman of the Bronx, electrolysist extraordinaire, taught me about the art of not tweezing, pointing out that if you tweeze a hair, the root becomes distorted, so that the electrolysis needle must go into that one hair root repeatedly until it is destroyed. So, dear ones, shave, cut or bleach, but don't tweeze.

The complaints at the opposite end of the spectrum are just as common: that of hair becoming thin. I hear my patients wail, "Brushfuls are coming out each day, going down the drain when I shower." Again, this is rarely a serious medical problem, but I do rule out thyroid imbalance and eating disorders. Then I look at dietary issues: most of us are deficient in the essential fatty acids that come from fish oils, flaxseed and primrose oil, all precursors to the building blocks of our steroid hormones.

A helpful combination of nutrients that I call my "baldness formula" includes Coenzyme Q10, biotin, copper, selenium, and zinc. It suggests washing the hair with a shampoo containing biotin, then rinsing with apple cider vinegar.

The most exciting thing I recently learned from my biochemist friend, David Zava, Ph.D., is that *saw palmetto*, the herb best known for prostate health, is remarkable for affecting hair to grow at the follicle level. I enticed a local compounding pharmacy to make a saw palmetto shampoo. I am now recommending it for my patients. None of these methods can harm, and, very possibly, they may help.

My wonderful Doctor of Pharmacy, Rebecca Cox, found a study of a mixture of saw palmetto, melatonin, and progesterone. She makes it into a cream that I instruct my patients to massage into their scalp, and with a shower cap left on throughout the night, this compound can invite the hair to grow at the follicle level.

Lastly, my Goddesses, always remember the body-mind-spirit connection. Ask yourself what stressors may be invading your life that might be taunting you with hair-raising issues. Remember that in certain cultures, hair is viewed as such a sensual adornment it is covered to all but the beloved one.

THE TRUTH ABOUT BUILDING STRONG BONES

Let's consider more deeply the bone protectiveness issue: remember how we have been hearing for years about the importance of estrogen in protecting us from osteoporosis. Indeed, estrogen has protective qualities—it prevents 50-60 percent of osteoporotic fractures—but let's put that into perspective.

To begin, we need a tiny anatomy lesson in bone metabolism. There are two components to healthy bone maintenance: (1) the osteoclast cells, or Pac-man munchers, as I call them, which devour old bone; (2) the osteoblast cells, which make new bones. Ideally, these two components are always in balance. And when they are, bone density remains stable.

But when osteoclasts outnumber osteoblasts, bone loss (commonly referred to as osteoporosis or bone thinning) occurs. Because estrogen is an osteoclast inhibitor, when a woman has too much estrogen, the breaking down of old bones, which is desirable, is inhibited.

Progesterone, on the other hand, is an osteoblast promoter, so, when utilized, bone mass actually can increase. And since there are absolutely no side effects to progesterone, a woman never has to feel pressured into stopping its use.

Surprising to many, by the way, is that the process of hormone imbalance starts as early as the mid-thirties, coinciding not-so-coincidentally with decreasing numbers of ovulatory menstrual cycles.

While we're on the subject of healthy bone mass maintenance, let's consider a larger picture. Losing bone is not only a hereditary phenomenon. It has as much to do with our lifestyles as with our family patterns. And this is where we can empower ourselves to control our destinies. There are four little habits that will mightily offend our bone density sensibilities:

- Smoking
- Alcohol abuse
- Animal fat consumption
- Daily doses of colas

Sadly, smoking and alcohol abuse often go hand in hand; we double our risk. Throw in heavy consumption of meat and dairy products, and we add another potent danger. Those of us naïve enough to believe the meat and dairy industries when they tell us that their products build strong teeth and bones need a brief lesson in biochemistry.

In Dr. Lee's outstanding book, *Natural Progesterone: The Multiple Roles of a Remarkable Hormone,* he explains that eating animal protein taxes the kidneys in their attempt to metabolize such protein. When taken in amounts exceeding bodily need, the urinary excretion of their waste products—uric acid and ammonia—causes a negative calcium balance. In other words, the excretion of calcium will exceed intake. This urinary loss of calcium would lower our blood calcium were it not for the parathyroid glands, which act to correct this serum deficiency by dissolving calcium from our bones to replace the loss. Get the picture? Robbing Peter to pay Paul here leads directly to osteoporosis.

It may be a shock to you to hear what an acceptable level of animal fat is, but here goes: more than two to four ounces of animal fat daily is harmful, especially if not organically farmed. And for those of us perpetually watching our waistlines, the kinder and healthier plant proteins in legumes and whole grains are the sensible, wholesome substitutes.

Our obsession with taking so many calcium tablets not only can cause constipation, but kidney stones, and calcifications in the joints and the breasts. We need to remember that vitamin D3, K2, magnesium, strontium, as well as trace minerals, are necessary for bone health.

The teaching that only weight bearing exercise builds bones becomes passé with the knowledge that frail, imbalanced women benefit from aqua aerobics.

A word about bisphosphonates, prescribed for osteoporosis and marketed as Fosamax, Actonel, and Boniva. These drugs have gotten a lot of bad press lately, for which I am grateful, because many women have such terrible digestive issues with these drugs. It is essential that you stand straight up, drink eight to sixteen ounces of water to be sure it washes down into the stomach. If it lodges in the esophagus, it can bore a hole in it. That is why you cannot lie down or exercise for one-half hour prior/after taking. One of my patients took her dose but dropped her car keys, bent over to pick them up and had burns in her mouth for two weeks!

Necrosis (death of) the jaw bone is also a real concern. Because these medicines have a very long presence in the body, as long as fifteen years according to Dr. Lee, the brittle quality of the bone persists. Remember, bone density machines are the gold standard to measure bone, but they are limited in that they measure *quantity* and not *quality* of the bone mass.

One last look at our standard American diet (SAD) finds an obsession with colas. These high phosphate drinks and other artificially carbonated beverages tend to increase bone loss of calcium.

We now know that bone healing can be inspired by energy medicine: a TENS unit[10] can be employed to encourage bone healing, as we must remember that it is living matter, and needs encouragement, as does a plant that thrives when it is prayed over.

Also, little known, but studied scientifically, is that the purring of a cat emits the identical frequency needed to heal bones! And the loving gaze of a kitten can heal on the spot!

---

[10] TENS unit is the acronym for **T**ranscutaneous **E**lectrical **N**erve **S**timulation. A TENS unit is a pocket size, portable, battery-operated device that sends electrical impulses to certain parts of the body.

Take Home Pearls

✧ See hot flashes as power surges, reminding the body that we are out of balance.

✧ Progesterone cream decreases hot flashes by almost 85 percent.

✧ Avoiding hot spicy food, alcohol, and caffeine help reduce flashes.

✧ Honor our needs with a good night's sleep, -preferably in a cooler room.

✧ For unwanted hair: bleach, trim, laser, electrolysis, but do not pluck.

✧ For thinning hair: essential fatty acids (fish oils, flax oil, coconut, olive, sesame, sunflower oils).

✧ Saw palmetto containing shampoos and creams grow hair at the follicle level.

✧ For bones, avoid colas, smoking, too much alcohol, excessive animal protein and the couch potato position.

✧ Don't just take calcium supplements which constipate: make sure they are balanced with magnesium and vitamin D3.

✧ Calcium rich foods best: salmon, sardines, almonds, green leafy vegetables, especially collards, kale, broccoli (crucifers) and carrot juice.

✧ Self love, taking our needs *first*, is key!

CHAPTER 6

Say Goodbye To PMS

All beliefs are illusions, so
you might as well choose healthy beliefs.
—Leonard Laskow, M.D.

A patient named Lorraine, whom I have known and loved since I came to the Lehigh Valley in 1990, visited my office for her yearly exam and proudly revealed to me that she finally stopped menstruating. At fifty-eight years old, she certainly had earned the right to "hold her blood," as our Native American sisters would say.

Lorraine's open disclosure prompted the confessional in me, and I was moved to relate a story to her that I'd told to frightfully few people. We hid in the examining room, me on my little stool, Lorraine perched on the tabletop and I started in.

Many decades ago when I was five years old, I accompanied Mom to the grocery store one sunny day while we were spending the weekend with her sister, my Aunt Mary, in South Jersey. Sent on a mission to retrieve a box of napkins, I proudly arrived back at my mother's side toting a box of Kotex. Mom blanched—there were men all around us in the store—and whispered, "No, Helene, those are not the right ones!"

"But Mom," I replied, "they're even better than napkins -- they're sanitary!"

Oh, how my mother blushed. The men within earshot snickered, and she came unglued, flustered to the hilt.

I was picking up the vibes but couldn't for the life of me figure out what was wrong. As I tugged on my mother with repeated pleadings to be enlightened, she tried to shush me, finally promising to speak to me when we got into the back of my cousin's pickup truck. Whereupon, I folded my arms across my chest and demanded, "Well?!"

That was when I learned about becoming a woman. But it wasn't until years later that I learned the secret of my mother's own dreadful experience upon entering womanhood. I have such love and compassion now for my mother just thinking about what she went through.

Mom was placed in an orphanage when she was a child. Having never been informed about how her body would be changing in adolescence or the facts about menstruation, at the first sign of blood, she feared she was dying and began to scream. But instead of comforting my mother and soothing her fears, the institution's matron gave her a beating for crying.

My dream for all young women who enter the hallowed sacred grounds of womanhood is that they be thrown a riotous party, to celebrate and pay tribute to this special occasion, so that they rise with pride to this new plateau in their lives. I feel the same way about menopause. It is the other end of this marvelous journey and should be celebrated with satisfaction and gratitude.

Pre-Menstrual Syndrome (PMS) is as much a part of the menopause cycle as are hot flashes. The term premenstrual tension has become a household word over the past several decades. It accounts for that out-of-body experience, or Dr. Jekyll-Ms. Hyde syndrome, that has our mates mystified and our children running for cover. The issue came to the fore in a big way years ago, when wide press was given to a case in England, where a woman was proclaimed "not guilty" in court because the murder she was accused of occurred during her premenstrual cycle.

Are premenstrual women raving maniacs?

And why do we not hear of PMS in other cultures?

Although a hard and fast biochemical cause cannot be ascribed to PMS, we do know that the one constant is its *cyclicity,* or the regularity with which it appears at a certain time in each menstrual cycle.

MOOD SWING MADNESS

Initially, when a woman first experiences PMS, she might complain of symptoms for three to four days prior to the menses. However, after a time, there often comes a sea of bad days, with only one symptom-free week. The following list, though only a partial one, reveals the diverse symptoms experienced by women suffering PMS: *abdominal bloating and cramping, fainting, hemorrhoids, asthma, back pain, breast swelling and pain, joint swelling and pain, insomnia, palpitations, food binges, fatigue, acne, aggression, confusion, salt and sweet craving, nausea, rage, sex drive changes, depression, swelling, herpes, hives, irritability, suicidal thoughts, lethargy alternating with increased energy, headaches, weight gain, lack of self-esteem and withdrawal from others.* In other words, PMS is an almost constant condition, with every imaginable symptom.

While much about PMS remains a mystery, we do know of its association with hormonal changes. Hormonal changes occur with the onset of menstruation for the first time, the few years preceding menopause, following the birth of a child, termination of a pregnancy, following the resumption of menses after a time of amenorrhea (no period), and, perhaps surprisingly, tubal ligation.

Many doctors today assure their patients, while preparing for tubal ligation, the surgical procedure that permanently ends fertility, that this simple surgery does nothing to alter hormone balance. Well, they are wrong. Dr. Lee found in the very hallowed scientific journal, *Obstetrics and Gynecology,* as long ago as 1979, a study that affirms a 50 percent reduction of progesterone in the women having their tubes severed over the control group not having the surgery! How's that for doctors not consulting their own literature!

WHERE'S THE CHOCOLATE?

Probably the most significant clue that PMS is rearing its head is what abides at the end of a fork. We know all too well how we dive into the chips and dips to satisfy our salt cravings, how we constantly fill up our coffee cups or open the soft drink cans in order to fix on caffeine. And let's not forget how we can empty a box of chocolates, though I can come to the defense of a small piece of dark organic chocolate, as it contains small amounts of magnesium and a substance called *ANANDA*-mide (which in Sanskirt means bliss), found to be a wonderful antioxidant. But by and large, these foods worsen our symptoms.

There is no doubt that the hormonal imbalance of too much estrogen is at play here. Studies have revealed that in women suffering PMS there is a lower than normal level of progesterone, thereby making the ten to fourteen days before the onset of bleeding actually estrogen-dominant. When we eat dairy products and red meat, we overload our systems with estrogen.

Remember, the petrochemicals in the air that get into the food chain add molecules identical to estrogen to the fat cells in our cows. And many of our animals are fattened with hormones, furthering the overwhelming quantity of estrogen in our bodies and affecting our PMS symptoms.

WHAT TO DO AND NOT TO DO

What are some treatments for this perplexing syndrome that is affecting more and more women in our high-tech, stressed-filled society? Well, I know of the treatments I would avoid because they are band-aid approaches and offer only a cover-up for symptoms rather than prevention.

Many caregivers prescribe diuretics, or water pills, in order to cause us to excrete excess fluid. But they abound with side effects: our kidneys are tricked into thinking that we are dehydrated, and a cascade of biochemical events occurs that often cause a dangerous imbalance of vital minerals in our system.

Prozac, marauding as Sarafem, is frequently prescribed for the one to two weeks before our periods, but these anti-depressants and anti-anxiety medications cover over the hormone imbalance and make us feel like zombies.

One of the first and most effective ways to change our PMS symptoms is with nutrition. Instead of a diet rich in refined sugar, caffeine, high fats and processed foods, let's get on a healthy bandwagon, embracing complex carbohydrates, whole grains, fresh vegetables and fruit, avoiding red meat and dairy products as much as possible, unless those dairy products are raw. This translates into thirty-five grams or less of fat per day and 75 percent of calories from complex carbohydrates. A high bean diet, especially hummus, lentil beans, baba ghonoush (egg plant), and lots of nuts, seeds and olives, sometimes referred to as the Mediterranean cuisine, is so healthy for us.

A noteworthy exception here relates to our sumptuously large sisters. High carbs don't always work for them because of an inability to metabolize them, a condition called insulin-resistance. They may best thrive on a high protein, low carb diet. And best we take half our proteins from fermented soy products and from plants, especially legumes. The other half can be organic meat, poultry and ocean fish.

The next order of business is exercise. The natural morphines (endorphins) released can give us such a feeling of well being, even when we prefer to roll up in the fetal position. These endorphins are optimal painkillers for the sometimes-dreadful dragging fullness and low back pain often experienced with our menses.

And since I am so excited about the availability of natural progesterone, let us not forget how helpful it can be during this time of hormone imbalance. When using the progesterone transdermal cream, I generally suggest one-quarter teaspoon twice daily, from ovulation until menses; for those of you not regularly ovulating (women as young as thirty-five and beyond), use it from right before symptoms begin until relief from symptoms occurs.

Lastly, some form of stress reduction is vital: prayer, meditation, yoga, and biofeedback. Get out in nature, listen to a beautiful symphony, read a book. PMS time is a time to "go inside" you. Listen to your quiet self. Love yourself.

Take Home Pearls

✧ Nutrition is key: avoiding sodas, refined sugars, too much caffeine; instead, snack on nuts, seeds, hummus, olives, as well as raw fruit and vegetables.

✧ Animal protein not organically farmed contains antibiotics and hormones, fueling PMS.

✧ Exercising five times weekly for twenty to thirty minutes releases natural morphine bubbles called endorphins to relax us.

✧ Natural progesterone balances excess estrogen and prevents PMS.

✧ Meditation and prayer are essential.

✧ Self love, taking our needs *first*, is key!

CHAPTER 7

Love Yourself &
Nurture Your Breasts

The secret of health for both mind and body is not
to mourn for the past, not
to worry about the future, or not
to anticipate troubles, but
to live the present moment wisely and earnestly.
—The Buddha

Now that you know me a little better, I can confess to you that while my love for healing has never waned, there was a time when I nearly severed my ties to the medical profession. My desire in this regard stemmed from two sources: the miserable, sleep-deprived "time I was serving" in medical internship and a budding relationship with a charismatic, sophisticated Brit, my soon-to-be second husband.

This alluring gentleman, several years older than I, who hailed from Hammersmith, England, arrived explosively into my life during my rotating internship. I first saw him exiting the train station sporting the traditional English umbrella and was delighted to learn that he lived right across the street. I learned that he ran a shipping line for a family-owned business based in Genoa, Italy. I was fascinated with him and schemed to meet him.

One day I dressed up coyly in a halter top and shorts and presented myself at his doorstep, cheekily asking if he would help me change the oil in my little red Mercury Zephyr. He showed obvious interest and happily consented to meet me in my driveway the next morning at ten.

Squeaky clean and impeccably made up, I presented myself at the appointed time. Ten o'clock came and went, as did eleven, then twelve. Frustrated and feeling rejected, I crawled under the car and in anger and released the oil cap, only to be splattered all over my carefully made up face with a flood of dirty oil.

Cleaned up and made up once again, I was sitting grumpily on my front porch reading the New York Times, when a car pulled up across the street. It was the Brit, Paul. I quickly covered my face with the newspaper and pretended to ignore him.

"Oh, hello," that limey voice melodically chimed. "Did you see my note?"

"What note?" I shot back arrogantly.

"Why, the note I left for you on my door," he explained.

"Look pal," I bellowed, "when you want to say something to someone in America, you leave a note on their door, not yours!"

Hands on hips, I marched across the street to have a look. His expertly scripted note asked for my forgiveness, for when he promised to assist me he had forgotten his commitment to play in a major golf tournament.

We were married seven weeks later, and the joy I took in Paul and this relationship was beyond my wildest dreams. He truly loved me and cared for me completely. My medical school-imposed financial worries were at an end, and I had a soul mate, confidante and playmate by my side, a dream come true.

Because my medical residency was so grueling and because I was now so happy, I intended to dump out of medicine. I was on my way to

tell my chairman he could "stick" his residency when the unbelievable
happened.

Paul's death left me devastated and inconsolable. I spent many nights wandering my apartment, martini in hand. I couldn't understand how God could take from me the only man I had ever truly loved and hadn't even given me a chance to say good-bye.

And then one night, my outlook changed. As I slept, Paul came to me, kissed me tenderly and said goodbye. My martini nights ended abruptly, and I soberly recognized that my pathway in medicine was to be steadfastly followed.

I had a flashback recently, after seeing a most magnificent, touching movie called *Life Is Beautiful*, about the horrors of the German concentration camps and one father's unconditional love, which somehow protected his young son from seeing man's inhumanity to man.

It was a flashback to 1962 when, as a second year student nurse, I greeted a new patient. Evelyn was forty-two years of age, a buxom redhead, who reminded me of Rita Hayworth. Evelyn's hair was a vibrant burnt orange shade of red, long and wavy, styled in a most fashionable beehive. Her lipstick had been patiently and perfectly painted on, and her full lips embraced the whitest, straightest teeth I had ever seen. She was, as I stretch my memory back, a bombshell. And I immediately loved her.

Evelyn entered the fourteen bed female ward fearful but filled with an offhand expectation that her illness was trivial and that soon, after some tests, she would be discharged.

I had no idea about what dreams Evelyn dreamt, but if she had them, they would be cut short, because she was to be delivered a death sentence. Diagnosis: invasive cervical cancer. Three months later, after a radical hysterectomy, a cystectomy--removal of the bladder with an opening through the skin of the abdomen for urine to drain, and removal of her sigmoid colon, with a colostomy providing yet another opening to the abdominal wall skin, this one draining bowel contents, she died.

Evelyn did not die with dignity. The surgery, dubbed a total exenteration, followed by radiation and chemotherapy, left her a mere skeleton with her once-magnificent red hair hanging limply and her sensual breasts now shriveled. The graphic depiction of the Holocaust in that film could only remind me of Evelyn.

Now, more than forty-five years later, still sad, I peruse the "what ifs?" What if Evelyn had known about the importance of yearly PAP smears? What if the sexual abuse she experienced at the hands of her father instead of being suppressed all those years had surfaced in time for her to have gotten counseling, so that she could release her anger and hurt and forgive her father. Perhaps her disease would not have expressed so virulently in her cell tissue. (Notice the direct correlation of the abuse to her diseased body organs.) With help, Evelyn might have been a gorgeous redheaded octogenarian today.

Having allowed myself this little reverie, I stand passionately in a quest to teach women how special they are. I urge women always to accept themselves exactly as they are and give themselves nurturing love and kindness.

When I was pregnant and living in Mississippi, I had a dream that revealed my mother had breast cancer. In my dream I made a vow to call the next day and urge my mother to see our family doctor. I suppose I suppressed the experience, because the promise I had made to myself came and went, and I didn't place that call. Two weeks later, my dream was to surface as reality, when Mom called to tell me that our family doctor had found a mass in her left breast.

Mindful of my dream and without skipping a beat, I charged right in, "Yes, Mom, and it's going to be cancer, but it will be all right." I then matter-of-factly began preparing my mother for what I knew would transpire: a modified, radical mastectomy with lymph node dissection, following which she would have to exercise her left arm to avoid what we call lymph edema, or swelling of the arm. I taught her over the telephone to practice movement by reaching up and combing her hair and walking up walls with her fingers.

Well, I was right! Mom's surgeon called, explaining that her lump had been a "garden variety" intraductal carcinoma of the breast with negative lymph nodes, meaning that the cancer was contained: it had not spread. She was fifty-eight years old and had been taking estrogen by itself for two years.

My mother survived the breast cancer, and later at the age of seventy-eight, she rallied over ovarian cancer.

TOO CLOSE FOR COMFORT

I now look at the many patients who are being diagnosed with breast cancer at a far younger age than my mother was: women in their late thirties and forties are being diagnosed with this devastating condition. I even know a very young woman, age twenty-five and pregnant with her first child, who has been given this dire diagnosis. What is this epidemic about and what can we do to prevent it?

There is no controversy that our stress-filled, joyless lives contribute to increased cancer in this land of ours. We are overburdened with work, overwhelmed with family care giving, over-committed to our families, professional groups and social schedules and over-run with high-tech toys. We frantically quest for what seems impossible: simple leisure time. And where do we find ourselves? *Depressed.* A surefire condition for lowering our immune systems.

Add to the equation our quick-fix foods that contain little or no nutritional value, and we set ourselves up for disease. I regularly say to my patients, "junk in, junk out," as I review their daily diets with them and note that we often treat our automobiles to better "food:" they get high-test gasoline, while we feed these sacred portals we call our bodies low-test, no-name fuel.

Chronic constipation, more common than we choose to acknowledge, is a major factor in promoting cancers of all kind, and I will devote in-depth discussion to this issue in Chapter 10.

And let's not forget about environmental toxins. One has only to look at the sharp rise in autoimmune diseases to know that the poisons in our air, land and water are playing havoc with our physical bodies. Xeno-estrogens are present in insecticides, herbicides and fertilizers. These "mimics of estrogen" that come from non-organic animal proteins (beef, pork, dairy products, poultry) attach to our fat cells and cause cancer, and the breast is particularly vulnerable.

We are so glib about what we use to contain our food and drink. Those flashy colored sport bottles and Styrofoam cups contain a deadly carcinogen, bisphenol A—a form of estrogen. Microwaving our food in plastics leech estrogen into our food. And microwave ovens change the molecular configuration of our food and emit dangerous electro-magnetic forces (EMFs).

The more we short change the magical symbiosis of our environment with our health, the more we introduce dis-ease and joylessness that prey into the hands of the medical soothsayers, who still say that disease is inevitable.

I have been measuring the vitamin D levels on all my patients, to find that ninety-eight out of one hundred women are deficient. We have been frightened out of the sun, and "the sunshine vitamin" is not only vital for bone health, it is also a pro-hormone that protects us from breast and colon cancer, as well as autoimmune illnesses, such as multiple sclerosis.

Because we are frightened out of the sun or told to use a high number sun screen, it and of itself is a carcinogen as it inhibits the healthy UVA rays as well as the UVB ones. Again, why not invite balance into our lives? Exposing ourselves to thirty minutes of sun daily before the hottest hours without sunscreen, and then covering ourselves with protective clothing or natural sunscreen made of herbs is wisdom.

IMPERFECTIONS AND INSECURITIES

Cosmopolitan Magazine did a study several years ago that questioned three hundred women about their breasts, how they liked the shape, the size, the placement and the configuration of their nipples. To a woman, each replied that she was unhappy with her breasts as they were. My sisters, listen up: we will never be free of breast cancer until we are free of the toxic belief that we are not good enough just as we are.

I had a personal revelation a few short years ago; it's one I might have come to much sooner. Born an only child, I was the classic people-pleaser. Since I had no siblings with whom to spar, I never learned how to defend myself when verbally or physically attacked. I wanted so desperately for everyone to love me that I played the court jester and buffoon with friends who were basically sallow and joyless. An excitement junkie, I was always pumping them up. It took over fifty years for me to *get it,* that during all these many long years of trying to win people over and gain their love, I was actually asking *me* to love *me*!

There is a virtue in selfishness. One of the many flaws in our thinking comes from our need to be loved. If we do what others ask or demand of us, and make them happy, surely they will love us. It is very common to see women, especially, feeling responsible for the home and hearth while our partners are out making a living—this was the old paradigm until women went back into the workplace in droves!

Our children, and now our parents—as we enter the sandwich generation—make unbelievable demands on us, and in our super-mode manner, we attempt to accomplish everything. The problem with this picture is that we do it, always deleting one major need: our own.

THOSE PESKY BREAST MACHINES

As long as I am into truth telling, I must go on record about my feelings regarding mammography. I was twenty-nine years of age when my mother was diagnosed with breast cancer. Recognizing the "family history" aspect of this disease, I began dutifully traipsing in for my yearly mammogram. I was a card-carrying believer in the benefits of mammography until recently when a quirky realization hit me square in the face: the mammogram results in no way assist us with prevention, do they? We may be able to diagnose breast cancer earlier, but it is still there. So many patients are sent back repeatedly for additional views and six month follow-ups for "stability" of a finding, that I am seriously concerned about the radiation that we are exposing our breasts to year after year. Granted, the doses are small, but they're also cumulative.

A BETTER WAY

There is a technique called *thermography* that deserves some serious attention here. Thermography is a diagnostic technique in which an infrared camera is used to measure temperature variations on the surface of the body, producing images that reveal sites of abnormal tissue growth. It can, without radiation, diagnose breast cancer. Fortunately, more and more women are seeking information about thermography. My colleague and friend, Phillip Getson, D.O., is a Cherry Hill, New Jersey, physician and authority on this safe, effective technique, and here are his words on the subject.

"First, some words on what we know now.

- *Breast thermography has increased eight fold in the past ten years.*
- *Seventy percent of all breast cancers are found on clinical self examination.*
- *The number one cause of breast cancer is radiation.*
- *Mammography has an inherent 15-20 percent false negative result.*

In the 1930's, a medical researcher warned the medical community about the dangers of compression of the breast for fear of spreading breast cancer.

None of these statistics are mine. They come from the American Cancer Association, the American Cancer Society, and other reputable organizations. They are startling to the point of being frightening. Why then do we, in America, limit ourselves to mammograms in patients forty years and older?

Indeed, why do we treat breast cancer retrospectively? We wait until a woman is diagnosed with breast cancer and then look for the most efficient treatment.

I have found that cancer is the only disease that we treat this way. After all, we take preventive measures to assure ourselves that we are in control of our diabetes, hypertension, heart disease, and cholesterol problems. In these instances, when there is a family history, we do careful monitoring before the problem occurs and adjust our diet, exercise, and life style.

However, with cancer, we wait until we get the disease and then we look for the best available treatment!

This, in my opinion, is unnecessary.

Thermography (or infrared imaging) actually predates mammography by almost a decade. The use of thermal imaging for non-medical reasons dates back to the Second World War and for medical applications to the mid-fifties. For many reasons, it has not achieved the widespread acceptance that other diagnostic tests have garnered. Nonetheless, it is a valuable diagnostic tool in the physician's armamentarium when properly used.

Thermography is a diagnostic test in which an individual stands two to three feet from an infrared camera which images the heat patterns of the breast transferring this information electronically to a laptop computer where highly sophisticated images are formed in color and black and white. This allows the interpreter to look at vascular patterns, their configuration and placement as well as heat patterns from one breast to the other to determine whether abnormalities exist of a physiologic nature. Whereas other tests, including mammography, ultrasound, and MRI are anatomic tests—they look for masses or lesions—Thermography is a physiologic study looking for changes in the activity of the breast to suggest abnormality.

It is well documented in medicine that changes in physiology predate the formation of anatomic ones. It has been shown in reputable research studies that physiologic changes in the breast can be found as much as seven to ten years before anatomic lesions can be seen on the aforementioned anatomic tests. This allows women to become proactive in their own breast health. They can then make changes in diet, nutrition, exercise, and life style that will minimize the likelihood of the formation of breast cancer by cutting off its sources of nutrients.

It has been shown that it is possible to forestall or even prevent the formation of cancer by making lifestyle changes.

Thermography is a simple non-painful, non-compressive, non-radiologic, diagnostic test that takes thirty minutes to complete. There is no risk. The images are easy to understand with some medical guidance which is provided.

Because of its non-invasive nature, it is not age dependent. It is available to women (and men) of any age.

We are not suggesting that Thermography should replace other testing. Certainly there is a need for both physiologic and anatomic study. It is however our mandate as physicians to provide our patients with the earliest (and least risky) means of diagnosis of any disease in order that treatment be initiated promptly and with the most benefit.

The study is cost effective when not covered by insurance. (Some insurers are re-imbursing for the procedure and some are not.)

This wonderful diagnostic screening procedure should be used by women of all ages to facilitate a proactive approach to health. Only by recognizing physiologic abnormalities at the earliest possible time, can we hope to correct them and maximize our health."

I advocate finding something safer and more effective than radiation. Aren't we worth it?

Breast cancer causes—environmental, hormonal, nutritional, and stress-related—can be changed with conscious, self-loving intention.

Take Home Pearls

✧ Pap smears save lives.

✧ Breast cancer can be prevented by attention to nutrition, environmental toxins, constipation, and hormonal balance.

✧ Thermography is a safe way to look at the *behavior* of breast tissue preceding tumors; whereas, mammography using radiation and compression can only address the *anatomy*, finding breast tumors long after they start.

✧ Self love, taking our needs *first*, is key!

Part II

Perfect Health:

A Birthright

CHAPTER 8

Let Food Be Your Medicine

I may not be perfect, but parts of me are excellent.
—Anonymous

I went to medical school in Mexico. For those of you who have bought into brainwashing that describes foreign medical students as inferior, let me enlighten you. First off, most of the schools abroad and those in Mexico have standards on a par with many of our schools back home. Though regulatory bodies differ in their stringencies, nonetheless, these foreign bastions of learning are not for the faint-hearted. For one thing, the lectures are all in that country's language, Spanish in my case. So are the exams. (Some of our more sadistic professors would confiscate question and answer books that we had brought from America to study for boards and have them translated into Spanish for us to sweat through.) And comparing notes with my colleagues in America fortunate enough not to ever have experienced Montezuma's revenge, I found that these spoon-fed students are handed study guides assisting them on what sections of the text to concentrate on. We, on the other hand, had to read the textbooks cover to cover. I actually read them three times, underlining and handwriting margin notes for emphasis. But these seeming difficulties were only minor inconveniences compared to some of the cultural differences I was fated to learn about.

Traditionally, I would return stateside for semester breaks and there I would hasten to work as an emergency room nurse to earn more living money. I would also take the courses not offered in Mexico that I would need for reentry into the American medical establishment.

One late night after returning to Mexico from one of these exhausting breaks and after a rocky ride from Mexico City to Tampico on a hair-raising puddle jumper, I arrived safely back, relieved and happy to be "home."

Or so I thought.

Arriving at Refugio's and Alex's home, I found it entirely vacant with no semblance of life of any kind. And no sign of my belongings.

"My bike, my books, my clothes!" I gasped, "Where is everyone? Where are my things?"

Confused, disheartened and clueless, I dragged myself to a hotel for the night. Early the next morning I returned to the scene, hoping against hope that life had returned to normal at my home away from home. As I approached, from out of nowhere a pleasant-faced man greeted me, "Elena?" (There is no "H" in Spanish pronunciation, so I became Elena."

"Si," I replied questioningly.

"Yo estoy Javier, y ahora viveras con nosotros." I was now to live with Javier, his wife, Alexandra, their son, Alex, and the family matriarch, Sra. Perez-Sanchez, Javier's mother.

I accompanied Javier to his home and lo and behold! found that all of my belongings had been moved out of my original home into theirs and put in exactly the same position that I had left them!

How this turn of events came to be I never found out. Refugio and Alex had my New Jersey telephone number. Why I might have expected a call from them, I can't imagine. I learned that other cultures often *have an interesting way of communicating.*

Javier's family and I would become very close. I was invited to their soccer games where they possessed a coveted season box; I danced at their parties while mariachi bands poured their hearts into their romantic music, and I attended the wedding of their daughter, Sylvia, a doctor in Mazatlan. What a glimpse into another culture and what an introduction to the notion that we Americans do not have all the answers.

I am Italian. That means I eat a lot of pasta. But in my home, growing up, it also meant eating lots and lots of sweets, because "sweets for the sweet" was our motto. My mother was a world-class chef, and I could always brag about a different scrumptious entrée each night of the week, except for perhaps one night when we would have a heated "leftovers" casserole, that in itself gourmet fare. My mother always taught me that casseroles taste better the second time, and to this day that conditioning holds.

Patrick Quillin, Ph.D., and Noreen Quillin write in their book, *Beating Cancer with Nutrition*: "The typical American is not in good health. Statistically speaking, the 'normal' American is overweight, lacking energy, constipated, mildly depressed, gets six colds per year and has dentures by age forty-five. Most develop obvious signs of chronic disease by their sixties, and die in their seventies from heart disease or cancer. Much of this deterioration in health comes from our diet.

"We are not destined to get sick and die young. We encourage this poor health through bad diet, lack of exercise, exposure to a wide array of toxins, and psychological stress."

Wow! I couldn't say it any better.

There is a different way to view the subject of food, different from the way we're all accustomed to thinking about it, and it involves more than simply taste. We need to consider what we eat, how we eat it, and we also need to be aware of how our food is grown.

THE MISERABLE REALITY OF OUR FOOD TODAY

When cows are locked in stalls, thanks to factory farms, injected with dangerous bovine growth hormone and antibiotics, these hapless animal brothers and sisters die in a short time, six to seven years instead of the twelve to sixteen year lifespan eating what God intended for them. The agribusiness factory farmers feed them candy bars and bakery scraps; when they lie dying, that is the meat we are sold for hamburgers.

There is a karmic issue here: we have been provided a vast wealth of animals and plants to feed these sacred portals called our bodies. When we eat from animals that have been tortured and imprisoned instead of permitting them to graze lazily on grass high in nutrients not poisoned with toxic chemicals, we assume in our bodies their suffering.

It is here that I would like to speak of the Weston Price Foundation. Dr. Price, a forward looking dentist, traveled around the world in the 1920s, and what he found was startling. When processed food—devoid of nutrients because of processed, simple sugars, touted as 'western commerce,' entered the diet of the worlds' peoples, he made an astonishing observation: the skull bones, round and generous, began to compress. The dental arches, heretofore sporting sixteen shiny teeth on top and sixteen on the bottom, were now pushed together, becoming filled with cavities as the bony arches narrowed. The once-happy smiles of Alaskan natives, having thrived on blubber and of the children in the Hebrides, who consumed raw dairy, lost their joy and healthy smiles when white flour and white sugar came insidiously into their diet.

Weston Price foundation groups have sprung up around the world affirming the life-saving effects of dairy and meat cows and poultry farmed as God intended: nibbling on grass and grains devoid of dangerous hormones and antibiotics.

Lest we fear raw dairy: let me remind you that in 1913 and 1927 in the respected medical journal, *Lancet*, it was stated that children drinking raw milk suffered much less from tuberculosis than those drinking pasteurized milk. In fact today, if you placed a virulent strain of the bacteria, E. coli, into pasteurized milk, it would thrive; if placed in raw milk with vitamins A and D and enzymes all intact, it would be destroyed soon after. Now, of course, you know that the American Dairy Association does not want you to know this, so I am telling you. An informed public is a healthy, empowered public.

A relatively high blood level of estrogen, resulting either from overproduction from these dietary sources or a decreased breakdown of estrogen in the liver continues unchecked when we further the insult by being vitamin deficient. When we are lacking in enough of the B vitamins, particularly B6, we are unable to inactivate estrogen in the liver.

Interestingly, vegetarians with a low fat, high fiber diet are known to excrete two to three times more estrogen in their feces than non-vegetarians. Other essential vitamins needed to metabolize estrogen properly are vitamins C, E, and the minerals, selenium and magnesium.

THIS DIET FOOLISHNESS

To begin, I want to loudly proclaim that *diets don't work*. They might seem to work for a while, but eventually our hand-to-mouth disease catches up, and all the reasons why we overeat come to the fore:

- we are bored
- we are scared
- we are nervous
- we are in a panic
- we are stressed
- we are angry
- we are lonely <u>and</u>
- we lack love

This last one is a biggie: *I lack love (ILL).* What does that really mean? That nobody loves us? No, it means that we don't love ourselves; therefore we cannot really love others, hence, we cannot receive love back.

Remember that infamous sixties-era grapefruit diet? How tedious, what deprivation! You can lose weight on that old grapefruit diet to be sure, but sustaining such a regimen is nigh on to impossible, and it won't be long before you're sinking your teeth into a big juicy steak and a pile of greasy French fries.

The Atkins diet has been around for a long while. I actually credit the good Dr. Atkins with some movement toward establishing a maintenance program, which introduces some carbohydrates after a heavy dose of protein and veggies.

Dr. Ornish's 10 percent fat diet made remarkable headlines

when he demonstrated that coronary artery blockage without surgery could be accomplished with his program of very low fat intake, moderate exercise, and a spiritual connection that might include prayer and meditation. This no doubt is one of the most balanced diet programs; however the lean to fat ratio is a bit stringent. Dr. Ornish does add essential fatty acids with Omega 3 and Omega 6 supplements, a positive additive because these healing fats are essential for life: they are building blocks for cholesterol, the precursor for sexual steroid production (without which little Johnnie doesn't get a baby sister).

Another diet program, this one to beware of: the *Carbohydrate Addicts Diet* allows a person for one hour of the day to pig out on any carbohydrate that is craved. So if eating four pounds of strawberry shortcake is your thing, you can go for it. I certainly can't imagine feeling very well or giving any stellar performances at any activity for the remaining twenty-three hours.

I could go on and on: there is the *Zone Diet*, and the *Eat for Your Blood Type* diet, both of which have downsides. The bottom line is that we need to learn to listen to ourselves, because our own inner voice will tell us what our bodies need.

THE CHOLESTEROL SHAM

This is probably as good a place as any to come to the defense of cholesterol. We have been duped by the American medical establishment and pharmaceutical industry (again) in regard to the cholesterol issue. They have attempted to intimidate us into believing that foods high in cholesterol, such as eggs, are bad for you. But eggs in fact are a perfect food, especially fertile, organic eggs. Other medical no-nos include shrimp, avocado, nuts, butter and other animal fats. But these, with the exception of non-organic animal fats, which are laced with antibiotics and hormones, are in fact very healthy foods.

We were duped into believing that the new-fangled vegetable oils like corn, canola and all those partially hydrogenated soybean products found in the processed foods we eat—chips, cookies, breads, cakes, and the like—are healthier than the natural fats found in organic meats, dairy and poultry. But these claims are bogus. Vegetable oils, particularly when they are heated, give off such dangerous amounts of hydrogenated toxins to our bodies that they are blowing holes in our arteries. Lard and mutton, dismissed as dangerous and causing heart disease, in fact, when eaten as organic meats and oil, can prevent heart disease.

My favorite healthy oils to cook with are extra virgin olive oil (never 'lite,' as all the dense nutrients become diluted), sesame oil, and organic coconut oil.

Cholesterol actually is the good guy: it's an antioxidant that attempts to patch these holes so that we don't die. Why our arteries eventually become clogged is because we continue our dietary indiscretions, such as gorging on rich sugar-filled, white flour desserts, that pollute our bodies.

We might note that prior to the sixties the medical establishment stated that a normal cholesterol level was 250. That level was dropped to 200. Could that possibly have been because the pharmaceutical companies developed cholesterol-lowering drugs that they couldn't wait to foist onto an awaiting public duped into thinking that they would save our lives?

The new lower total cholesterol and low density lipoproteins (LDL) evokes fear in my heart. We need cholesterol to be the precursor of all our sex steroids, which include progesterone, testosterone, estrogen, and cortisol. When we lower the total cholesterol too far down (I think 150 is *too* low), we are seeing higher levels of aggressive behavior, depression, suicide, and cancer. Moreover, cholesterol lowering drugs, such as Lipitor, cause the destruction of the myelin sheaths covering our nerve cells (neurons), and we are becoming forgetful and demented earlier. I cannot help but wonder if the epidemic of Alzheimer's disease is in part caused by such low cholesterol levels. A brother to Lipitor, Baycol, was taken off the market after fifty people died of rhabdomyelosis, destruction of muscle cells, the most important becoming the heart muscle. And it inhibits the synthesis of coenzyme q10, a great heart healthy nutrient.

This is where I stand on meat and dairy products: for my patients, who are seriously ill, particularly with cancer. I always nudge them into forgoing meat, dairy and poultry while they are healing. Those products are so difficult to metabolize that the body becomes overtaxed trying to digest them, and there is little energy left over that the body can devote to getting well. But for the healthy person, who feels better eating animal protein, be sure you are putting into your system *organic meat, poultry, pork, and raw dairy products.*

SUGAR BLUES

A wonderful book by William Dufty, *Sugar Blues*, gives a sobering account of our illustrious history of sugar consumption in this country. At the turn into the twentieth century, we were each consuming about one to two pounds of sugar each year. That number has increased to a shocking and unbelievable one hundred to three hundred pounds of sugar per person per year! Do you wonder why we have so much obesity, diabetes, heart disease, cancer, fibromyalgia, with such an imbalance in our diet?

WHAT'S WRONG WITH EATING RIGHT?

Our justification for not eating healthy is that healthy food doesn't taste good, but this is a cop-out. There are many, many delicious vegetarian dishes being taught in nutrition classes, on TV programs, and available in a myriad of cookbooks. Many diets have been developed by visionaries such as Kushi, Gerson, Christopher, who have all been instrumental in helping to reverse degenerative diseases. Though they have varying philosophies, they nonetheless adhere to the following food basics:

> They use only unprocessed food.
> They use only fresh vegetables organically grown.
> They employ a low-fat diet.
> They emphasize the importance of bowel regularity.
> They use few or no dairy products, with yogurt the preferred dairy selection, and preferably raw.
> They stabilize blood sugar levels with no sweets, and rarely eat something sweet by itself, if in fact sweets are eaten.
> They increase potassium and reduce sodium intake.
> They stress frequent, small meals.

LESSER-USED BUT MIGHTY-HEALTHY APPROACHES TO FOOD

- The macrobiotic methodology, employing beans, grains, fruits, shoots, and lots of vegetables, has been scientifically proved to prevent and heal cancer. I practiced this diet for ten years and had vibrant health—and some of the most amazing bowel movements—and still incorporate it into my eating at times. The Weston Price Foundation—affirming the healing qualities of raw dairy and meat and poultry and pork grown sustainably as God would have it—has healed many illnesses. And this foundation, as Michio Kushi, who brought the macrobiotic diet into American thought, adheres to the importance of eating from under your own tree: that is, eating foods in season instead of trucking them thousands of miles, worsening global warming and increasing carbon use.

The healing macrobiotic diet increases one's variety of food selections, eating regularly and in less quantities and maintaining an active, positive life and mental outlook. It has brought many who have followed its teachings back from the brink of death. However, strict followers sometimes find this diet most restrictive. And some people are put off by it because meals take a great deal of time to prepare.

- Raw foodists will teach with passion that cooking your food destroys vital nutrients. **Raw foodism** is a lifestyle promoting the consumption of uncooked, unprocessed, organic foods as a large percentage of the diet. Raw foodists typically believe that the greater the percentage of raw food in the diet, the greater the health benefits. They claim that raw food encourages weight loss and prevents and/or heals many forms of illness and chronic diseases. This is a time intensive diet and one that I personally with my lifestyle could not honor, but truly eating at least 30 percent of our food raw in salads, nuts, seeds will be beneficial in many ways.

MY OWN PERSONAL FOOD FARE

I used to think that couscous, kashi, millet, and bulgur were provinces in the Sudan and that adzuki, garbanzo and pintos were horses instead of beans. But you know what? I began macrobiotics and it took me only three weeks to develop new, healthy eating habits, and you can do it too!

I tend to be a very modified macro lover. I am a fish vegetarian—mostly. I eat some form of beans, whole grains, and fresh vegetables each day. But I love fish and will indulge in a good piece of salmon and/or shrimps weekly. And never think me stodgy: once in a while I indulge all my senses in a slice of my beloved pepperoni pizza or a burnt hot dog with all the trimmings.

My bow to the raw foodists comes in the form of breakfast. Daily I concoct a blender drink of dehydrated organic foods[11] mixed with Udo's blend of sunflower, evening primrose, coconut, sesame and flaxseed oils. I add to it cod liver oil[12], ground flaxseeds, which contain lignans[13], juice, banana, shredded coconut, and blueberries. This she-woman drink provides most of my nutrients.

THE BADLY-RAPPED BEAN

I have grown to love beans. They have been given a bad rap because everyone thinks they make you fart, and actually they do when you first change your diet from high meat and dairy to macrobiotic like I did. You can minimize gas by soaking the beans overnight in water, then throwing away that water and cooking them in fresh water. Adding a piece of sea vegetable, such as Kombu, found in your health food store is a further help.

Beans are delicious, nutritious and a rich protein source for the vegetarian. They are a major component of the macrobiotic diet.

THE FRAGRANT FLOWER - GARLIC

Where do I start with this remarkable food? Its use can be traced back to the cave man. Remains of this odiferous herb have

---

[11] My wonderful friend, Tom Maslar, a fellow herbalist, makes a powder called Nature's Greens. His company is called *Apollo Nutrition*.
[12] *Nordic Naturals* is my favorite.
[13] Lignans bind excess estrogen and help prevent estrogen-fueled cancers, such as breast and uterine.

been found in caves inhabited ten thousand years ago. It was found in the tomb of King Tut. And do you know that fifteen pounds of garlic once bought a healthy male slave?

The pungent odor of garlic, which is both loved and loathed, is caused by the sulphur compound, *allicin,* which is responsible for its potent health benefits. Louis Pasteur was the first in 1858 to prove that garlic was an antibiotic. He demonstrated how it could kill bacteria in laboratory culture dishes.

Besides its heart healthy qualities, which we will get to momentarily, multiple studies have confirmed that garlic is effective not only against bacteria, yeasts, and fungi, but against parasites and even viruses. Candida fungus and the herpes virus are but two for which garlic can be used.

When it comes to heart health, studies have shown that when garlic is consumed with a fatty meal, the resulting level of fats and cholesterol in the blood is dramatically reduced. In fact, taking this popular herb for a couple of months can reduce the level of blood cholesterol by 15 percent, even more if combined with a proper diet. When taken regularly, garlic significantly reduces the LDL (bad cholesterol) and raises the HDL (good cholesterol), as well as protecting against the plaque that hardens the arteries and subsequently causes blockages.

Very importantly, in addition to lowering blood fats, garlic has anti-platelet activity. In other words, it inhibits clotting. This blood "thinning" effect reduces the risk of strokes and heart attacks. Garlic also lowers blood pressure.

A confounding practice of doctors who give patients prescriptions for blood-thinning drugs is to warn them against garlic and the cancer-protecting cruciferous vegetables, such as broccoli, kale, cauliflower, brussel sprouts, because they contain coumarins, which are blood-thinners. My rhetorical question is *why not allow the patients to have the healing foods and lower the dose of risky blood thinners?*

A cancer researcher working at Sloan Kettering Hospital in New York City demonstrated that garlic, the humble smelling rose, could actually inhibit the growth of cancer cells. And do you know what Sloan Kettering did with him? They fired him. Surprised? Well, don't be. You must know by now that our conventional medical system has not yet broken bread with the idea that natural healing is as powerful a modality as it is and at a fraction of the cost. One of my brilliant teachers, Dr. Richard Schultze, adds garlic to many of his herbal tinctures, rendering them more potent than most on the market. He also encourages fresh raw garlic in the daily diet. Because many of us worry about bad breath, we often substitute garlic tablets, but the pills are a weak second choice. They simply don't have the potency of fresh garlic. You can chew fresh parsley or suck on some roasted coffee grounds for fresher breath; better yet, share it with your loved ones!

To illustrate the power of the healing protectiveness of garlic, let me share a story about four French thieves who survived Bubonic Plague several centuries ago. The king promised these thieves that he would spare their lives if they would explain how they could steal gold fillings from the mouths of infectious corpses without contracting the disease. The answer, my friends: you guessed it— garlic! They apparently drank garlic juice and also soaked the bandanas they wore over their nose and mouth with a mixture of garlic juice and other herbs. Food for thought! I suppose soon the question will be not whether you keep garlic in your house, but *where,* in the kitchen or the medicine cabinet.

THE BIG THREE

Here are my favorite healing foods:

1. Yogurt. It contains the active culture of bacteria called Lactobacillus, which can actually fortify the immune system. Besides tripling the amount of Interferon—a powerful immune system weapon that kills cancer cells—it has also been shown to slow down the growth of tumor cells in the GI tract. By the way, I do not refer to the sugar-filled varieties found on most market shelves. Plain organic yogurt is delicious all by itself. If you like, though, you can add your own fresh fruit to top it off. Raw organic yogurt is best.

2. Garlic. You know about this guy already.

3. Cruciferous vegetables. These include kale, broccoli, cabbage, brussel sprouts, and cauliflower. These contain indoles, a phyto-chemical that appears to be protective against cancer.

A CARROT BY ANY OTHER NAME . . .

The story of organic produce is valid and, thankfully, growing. The recent promotion of organic foods is not moneymaking hype. The concept is about the serious business of bringing us back to the perfect health God intended for us to have.

We have raped our land in the name of profit. Instead of letting our fields lie fallow for the time it takes to permit valuable nutrients to replenish themselves, we add to it noxious fertilizers and insecticides that are filled with xeno-estrogen compounds. These additives poison our food stores, particularly our animal and dairy stocks whose fat components have an affinity for the fat-soluble hormones.

Several studies have been performed showing the marked increase in minerals and vitamins in foods grown organically versus those grown conventionally. Here is a summary of a Rutgers

University Study comparing nutrients in commercially grown, inorganic vegetables with organic vegetables grown in naturally fertilized soil:

	Percentage of Dry Weight		Millequivalents per 100 Grams of Dry Weight				Trace Elements in Parts Per Million (Dry Matter)				
	Total Ash or Mineral Matter	Phosphorus	Calcium	Magnesium	Potassium	Sodium	Boron	Manganese	Iron	Copper	Cobalt
SNAP BEANS											
Organic	10.45	0.36	40.5	60.0	99.7	8.6	73	60	227	69	.26
Inorganic	4.04	0.22	15.5	14.8	29.1	0.0	10	2	10	30	00
CABBAGE											
Organic	10.38	0.38	60.0	43.6	148.3	20.4	42	13	94	48	.15
Inorganic	6.12	0.18	17.5	15.6	53.7	0.8	7	2	20	.04	00
LETTUCE											
Organic	24.48	0.43	71.0	49.3	176.5	12.2	37	169	516	60	.19
Inorganic	7.01	0.22	16.0	13.1	53.7	0.8	6	1	9	3	00
TOMATOES											
Organic	14.20	0.35	96.0	203.9	257.0	69.5	36	68	1938	53	.63
Inorganic	6.07	0.16	47.5	46.9	84.6	0.8	5	1	1	0	00
SPINACH											
Organic	28.56	0.52	96.0	203.9	257.0	69.5	88	117	1584	32	.25
Inorganic	12.38	0.27	47.5	46.9	84.6	0.8	12	1	19	0.5	.20

Rutgers University concluded that commercially grown inorganic vegetables are very low in mineral and trace mineral content.

And, to be sure, organic foods taste better. I strongly suggest you seek out local organic farmers who respect and love their land instead of buying produce grown joylessly by our megalithic agribusiness corporations.

HEART HEALTHY NUTRIENTS

Here are two more:

1. Coenzyme Q10 (Ubiquinone)

    It is a given that every cell in our body needs energy to function optimally. One nutrient that appears to have the universal effect of promoting greater cellular energy and longer life is CoQl0. It is often referred to as the universal energy molecule, probably because its other name is ubiquinone, from which the word *ubiquitous* comes. A past issue of *Nutrition News* notes: "Studies have shown that if levels of CoQ10 decline to a 25 percent deficiency, our organs and systems cannot meet their energy requirements ... below a 75 percent deficiency, life can no longer be sustained." People on cholesterol lowering drugs, such as Lipitor, Provachol and Zocor, need to supplement with Q10 because these drugs lower the body's level of this necessary nutrient.

2. L-carnitine

    This is a very special amino acid, or "building block" of proteins. And remember, proteins are essential in providing the structure of all living things. In the human body, protein substances make up the muscles, ligaments, tendons, organs, glands, nails, hair, and body fluid. Next to water, protein makes up the greatest portion of our body weight. There are approximately twenty-nine commonly known amino acids that account for the hundreds of different types of proteins present in all living things. L-carnitine is biosynthesized in the liver and is found in highest concentration in muscle and organ meats in our diet; interestingly, it is not found in vegetable sources.

Using carnitine as a food supplement can encourage appropriate metabolism of fats and prevent ketosis. This can be an important addition to a *sensible* weight loss program.

VITAMINS & MINERALS FOR VITALITY

It is said that when we first came to this wonderful country almost four hundred years ago, there was sixty feet of topsoil. We are now down to four to six inches! Let me explain what this means in terms of the nutritious quality of our food. In 1948 three ounces of spinach contained 158 milligrams iron; in 1973, it was down to 27 milligrams; in 1986, 2 milligrams. A study done by the Rutgers University assayed the vitamin and mineral content of an organically grown tomato and one conventionally grown (see table). The organic tomato contained almost twice the nutrient value. Am I clearing the picture for you? Well, what does it mean in practical terms? Let's put it this way: you would never put sugar in your gas tank and expect your car to run, would you?"

An amusing but sad sign hangs on the cages of our zoo animals: "Do not feed the animals human food: it could kill them."

There has been a common theme about vitamins in the medical profession: if you eat a healthy and balanced diet, you don't need vitamins. But I will tell you, not only is our soil almost completely depleted of nutrients, we have to couple that with rampant pesticide and herbicide usages, and residues from other toxic substances, such as DDT. Indeed, we are deficient in many needed vitamins and minerals.

Walking into a pharmacy or health food store can be a sensory overload experience. What product to buy? Every employee will have his or her favorites, either from experience or vested interest.

Most importantly, it is necessary for you to know the difference between *natural and synthetic* supplements. Many of our vitamin and mineral products are mass-produced by large pharmaceuticals, and they put in them sewer sludge, ground up oyster shells, even animal feces (and they call these *natural ingredients)*. At best these products are useless, at worst, harmful, but no matter which, our bodies cannot assimilate them. Consider Vitamin B12 for a moment: the synthetic is made with the chemical *cyanocobolamin,* the natural with bluegreen algae, spirulina. Which do you think is the best one?

Be sure that your vitamins and minerals are made from food sources and not toxic petrochemicals.

I'll end this chapter with some pearls of wisdom that I have come to treasure:

- Have a love affair with your food.

- Be in the moment with your food. Savor the taste and aroma. And don't do anything else while you're dining. Painting toe nails, answering your email, talking on the telephone, and teaching your teenager about safe sex doesn't make for good digestion

- Prepare only whole, live food, not dead, denatured, fake food.

- Know food as your friend, not the enemy that is sure to add a bulge to your thighs.

Take Home Pearls

✧ Diets don't work, healthy eating does.

✧ When at all possible, consume animal proteins without antibiotics and hormones.

✧ Eat locally grown food to avoid further taxing our environment.

✧ Garlic protects us from viral, bacterial, and fungal infections, and is very heart healthy.

✧ Organic food has more nutrients than non-organically grown food.

✧ Self love, taking our needs *first*, is key!

CHAPTER 9

Nightmare on Nutrastreet

The physician is sent to entertain the patient while
God does the healing.
—Albert Schweitzer

During my early years at Jersey City Medical Center, the bulk of my patient load was the clinic patients who had multiple challenges, mostly with high-risk pregnancies. Few private patients came to this large, MASH-unit-like hospital: crossing through the indigent housing projects nearby could be fraught with danger. Occasionally, I cared for a private patient, who was usually part of our own medical or nursing staff.

Susan was one such patient, the head nurse in our gynecology unit. In her late forties, Susan had stopped her menses several years earlier, her early menopause likely a result of having had her tubes tied and also being a heavy smoker. She confided to me that she was spotting.

I arranged for Susan to come to my private consultation suite where I examined her and performed an endometrial biopsy, a procedure somewhat like a D and C. My heart sank as I felt her uterus: it was rock-hard and unusually large, bigger than a football. I dreaded the biopsy results, and what I feared proved true: cancer, on the move, growing aggressively.

An extensive workup ensued, and finally my gynecological oncologist and I operated on her. She had a rare but virulent type of sarcoma. Her prognosis was poor. All that was available to her was chemotherapy, yet this too would provide only a dismal outlook.

Susan was a trooper, and when all her hair fell out, she wore a stylish bandana when she came for treatment. I would close the door and hold her hand, hugging her frequently as we strove to mastermind through some strategies to ease her pain and nausea. What was so agonizing for me was that I was in a profound, debilitating depression, and my own pain was psychically paralleling Susan's. Helping her was a major struggle, as I could barely stay afloat myself.

Six months into her disease, she lapsed into a light coma, rousing only briefly when she heard her name.

So much pain surrounded this woman: divorced from her cardiologist husband and estranged from her daughter, she had very little emotional support.

My chief resident was intently following her case. Even though her prognosis was so very poor, he proceeded to write orders for a full resuscitation if her heart stopped beating.

After Susan had been in a coma for several days, obviously in a terminal state, I walked into her room, held her hand, kissed her lightly on her forehead and whispered that it was all right to let go. She died peaceably an hour later, after I saw to it that no bells rang or whistles blew to signal that machines of indignity should be brought in to assault her.

When my chief resident found out, he berated me for not attempting to resuscitate Susan, despite the fact that she was terminally ill and in interminable pain.

Sometimes we doctors see death as our own personal failure. Unfortunately, we suffer from the illusion that we are in charge of life and death. I try to remember the arrogance of such an attitude and remember too that I am God's servant in a scheme of things that is much larger than I can see.

After I began practicing medicine, it didn't take me long to see, truly realize, how intensely and completely we can abuse our bodies and our minds. The constant, repetitive stream of patients with chronic, multiple complaints of illness into my office was evidence of that.

When a patient arrives with symptoms, a good doctor rules out all the medical possibilities—tumors, metabolic illnesses, hormonal imbalances—first before going on to look for emotional issues that can expose our immune states to illness. (Finally, I am getting more comfortable with challenging the status quo, the norm that conventional healers accept as okay.)

One of my patients, a healthy sixty-three year old woman, whom I have known for five years, came in to visit and reported that she had just been diagnosed with multiple sclerosis. I asked my usual, standard questions, then played a hunch: "By any chance, do you use any NutraSweet products?"

"Oh, well, my dear, I drink six cans of diet Pepsi every day and have done so for many years!"

Back in 1965 a chemist working for G.D. Searle, the pharmaceutical company, accidentally discovered aspartame while testing an anti-ulcer drug. In 1983, over the objection of many scientific investigators, the FDA approved aspartame as an artificial sweetener to be included in carbonated beverages.

Actually, what started my curiosity about the safety of aspartame, branded NutraSweet, was a story by one of my patients about her husband's hospitalization for a grand mal seizure. Routine investigations were undertaken, looking for brain tumors, infections of the spinal cord and meninges (covering of the brain and spinal cord), along with infectious or metabolic causes that might be responsible for the convulsion. All testing results showed up negative. Finally, what surfaced was that this man with daily regularity was drinking three to four cans of diet soda!

FRIGHTENING FACTS

This fact piqued my curiosity, and I sent my son on an Internet search. The results of his research shocked me. Aspartame is comprised of three chemicals: aspartic acid, phenylalanine, and methanol.

Let's start with methanol: methanol is a wood alcohol, a deadly poison. You have only to think of the skid row alcoholic who winds up blind or dead to get a vivid picture of what ingesting this lethal toxin does.

Methanol is gradually released in the small intestine when the methyl group of aspartame encounters the enzyme chymotrypsin. The absorption of methanol into the body speeds up considerably when free methanol is ingested, this being created when aspartame is heated above eighty-six degrees Fahrenheit. Remember all the illness reported by our soldiers returning from the Gulf War? They consumed thousands of cans of diet soda, which sat in the blazing sun. And what about diet Jell-O, as we heat it to boiling prior to cooling?

Methanol breaks down into formic acid, the venom put out by an ant when it stings; formaldehyde, a neurotoxin used as embalming fluid; and diketopiperazine (DKP), a byproduct of aspartame, which causes brain tumors in animals. The EPA recommends a limited consumption of methanol to 7.8 milligrams per day. A one-liter (approximately one quart) aspartame sweetened beverage contains about fifty-six milligrams of methanol. It is not uncommon for some of us addicted to soda to consume 250 milligrams of methanol daily, greater than thirty-two times the EPA limit!

Some of the symptoms of methanol poisoning include: headaches, buzzing in the ear (tinnitus), dizziness, nausea, gastrointestinal disturbances, weakness, vertigo, chills, memory lapses, numbness, shooting pains in the extremities, behavioral disturbances, and neuritis. The most well known problems from methanol poisoning are vision problems including misty vision, progressive contraction of visual fields, blurring of vision, retinal damage, and blindness.

Formaldehyde is a known carcinogen: it causes retinal damage, interferes with new cell growth, and causes birth defects. Since we humans lack a number of key enzymes that help to speed up metabolic functions, we are actually much more sensitive to the toxic effects of methanol than are animals.

NutraSweet also contains aspartate, or aspartic acid. This is an amino acid that we know acts as a neurotransmitter, which facilitates transmission of information from one neuron to another in the brain. When there is too much aspartate, brain cells are killed off because too much calcium is going into those cells. In excess, aspartate is referred to as an "excitotoxin" because it excites the neural cells ... to death. Many chronic illnesses are affected negatively by long term exposure to this excitatory amino acid, among them: multiple sclerosis (MS), Lou Gehrig's Syndrome (ALS), memory loss, epilepsy, Parkinson's disease, AIDS, dementia, Alzheimer's disease, Lupus, Lyme's disease, fibromyalgia.

The final ingredient of aspartame, phenylalanine, also an amino acid, may be known better if I remind you of the "heel stick" given to your newborn baby. This is a test for a rare genetic disorder called phenylketonuria (PKU), in which the body cannot metabolize phenylalanine. This condition leads to often-lethal doses of this substance in the brain. Studies have shown that ingesting large amounts of aspartame, even in those without this rare disorder, can cause dangerously high levels of phenylalanine in the blood. Excessive levels in the brain can cause serotonin levels to decrease, leading to emotional disorders such as depression.

H. J. Roberts, M.D., a diabetic specialist and leading pioneer in the investigation of aspartame dangers, has revealed that the American Diabetes Association (ADA) recommends NutraSweet as an artificial sweetener despite the following: (1) it can precipitate clinical diabetes; (2) it causes poorer diabetic control in diabetics on insulin or oral drugs; (3) it leads to aggravation of diabetic complications such as retinopathy, cataracts, neuropathy, and impairment of the digestive tract; (4) and finally, it can cause convulsions.

Overall toxicity from the use of aspartame includes the following symptoms: tremors, slurred speech, confusion, chronic fatigue, depression, irritability, panic attacks, marked personality changes, phobias, tachycardia (rapid heart rate), chest pains, high blood pressure, diarrhea, abdominal pain, itching, menstrual problems, weight gain, hair loss or hair thinning, joint pains, headaches, bloating.

Since we are seeing NutraSweet in more and more products, its implication for illness grows.

Why when we have stevia and some newly investigated sugars—xylitol—must we continue to use such a toxic substance. It is sadly rhetorical because the moneymakers have deigned it so, and we have remained lobotomized and buy into the mistruths.

Take Home Pearls

✧ Aspartame (Nutrasweet) is a neurotoxin and should be banned from use!

✧ Nutrasweet causes seizures, headaches, and keeps weight glued to our bodies.

✧ Natural sweeteners, xylitol and stevia are safe, and tasty.

✧ Splenda contains a chlorine molecule which is not healthy for us.

✧ Self love, taking our needs *first*, is key!

CHAPTER 10

Constipation Kills

My barn having burned to the ground,
I can now see the moon.
—Taoist saying

As a medical student in Mexico, I liked to ride my bike down the main street of Tampico. One day I was stopped at a red light. At the signal's change I proceeded to cross the street. But so did a VW bug coming from the other direction. Before I knew what was happening I was sailing into the air, then crash landing onto my backside, with a crack on the head thrown in for good measure. All I remember is the blood and the paralysis in my toes. In my pain all I could think was, Dear God, please if I am going to die, let it be in New Jersey where I was born.

Needless to say, I was terrified: here I was a Gringo in a foreign land, not so fluent in Spanish. How would I get help?

Suddenly, from out of nowhere a man scooped me into his arms, and plopped me onto the back seat of a taxi. My savior delivered me to a Red Cross Hospital, presumably in the emergency room where I was rudely dumped onto a cold slab-like table.. An insolent nurse arrived, hurling a suspicious, insensitive query, "Que paso a te?" (What happened to you?), whereupon she proceeded to shave my treasured tresses surrounding my head wound. Next, she came at me with a huge syringe and before I had a chance to holler, she stuck that needle into my butt and pushed in an ominous fluid. Then another strong set of arms was lifting me onto a litter and shoving me into an ancient ambulance. With a sudden lurch the maniacal driver took off. The back door flew open and the litter I was strapped to began rolling toward the open door. Desperately, I flung out my arms to stop myself from flying out.

Finally, we arrived at our destination, my medical school hospital, where I was unloaded onto another cold slab. My head wound was sutured with what felt like a thick piece of rope. Then I was carted off to a room, occupied this night by a bevy of flying animals, that included giant mosquitoes, bats and beetles, for, you see, there were no window panes. An IV was started, and strange people arrived periodically to knock on my knees, tickle my feet and shine light in my eyes, checking to see whether I was still alive.

I didn't have to wait long for the real trouble to begin: an officious nurse with another huge syringe loomed over me, and before I could ask what she had in it, she jabbed me, injecting the contents at rapid speed. Suddenly, my eyes saw black and my ears buzzed with pressure: I felt like I was in a wind tunnel and truly thought I was dying.

So what did I do?

I did what any normal red-blooded American female would have done: I screamed bloody murder. What I later found out was that the syringes contained Decadron, a potent cortisone drug. And I had been given nearly five times the safe dosage.

Finally, after a nightmarish eighteen hours, a radiologist x-rayed my back, and we discovered I had a separation in the sacroiliac joint, an injury, which still gives me daily reminders of that loathsome experience.

Frustrated, beaten and in pain, I flew home for R & R and some

precious days with my family. I took anti-inflammatory drugs (Motrin)
to numb the soreness, but unfortunately, it also gave me gastritis.

It's odd that that experience didn't cause me to flee to some other way of practicing medicine—perhaps to the witch doctors in Africa—but it wasn't until years later, close to my fiftieth birthday, when I met a chiropractor, whose skilled hands changed the way I viewed alternative medicine, that my journey into healing truly commenced.

From early childhood, bowel movements were for me a chore. It was the forties, and although Hippocrates had been around for millennia touting my oft quoted, "Let food be your medicine and medicine be your food," I preferred the bulk after and before meals to be candy. Remember those varicolored little bumplets that came stuck on that long narrow paper resembling adding machine tape? Well, my buddies and I would go to the corner apothecary and spend our pennies on those little beauties, as well as on Jujubes, Snickers, Milky Way, and Mounds Bars. I was, I think, the first to understand the meaning of "life's too short: eat dessert first!"

Eating sugar all day long didn't leave much room for anything else other than those wonderful home-cooked meals Mom made, like drinking lots of water or exercising. So what else could I do but dutifully take the ExLax or Milk of Magnesia.

Remember when you were a small child and your mother would praise you for the mammoth poop that you so proudly displayed in the toilet? What happened to the glee of such life-affirming simplicity? Well, we grew up. And all our joyful spontaneity went with it. It is no longer fashionable to talk about excrement once we leave our youth and become sophisticated adults. And we would never want to admit any connection with the metaphysical understanding: that constipation represents a resistance to change and persistence in living old habits and old thought processes.

A SUBJECT TO AVOID?

When I used to ask my patients, "and how are your bowels?", they would answer "fine." I wised up fast. I realized that "fine" could mean anything from a daily bowel movement to one once a week or even as rarely as twice a month. Now I ask "how often?"

You know those little hard pellets that you pass that resemble gerbil food? Well, those little pellets are an indication that your body is toxic: they can be why you are depressed, fatigued, have brain fog, heavy bleeding, endometriosis, fibroids in your uterus and cysts in your breasts. And all of these conditions have one major excess in common: estrogen.

When we do not properly excrete our foods, and remember, by the way, that they contain xeno-estrogens from the petrochemicals used as insecticides and fertilizers, we reabsorb them, and they poison us.

Healthy people poop after every meal. And the stool is light brown in color and breaks up easily in the water. Dark or marbled stools indicate you are eating too much fat. Same thing goes for stool that sinks like the Titanic or those that float.

One of the greatest healers on the planet today (and also my beloved teacher—remember him from Chapter 6?) is Richard Schultze, a naturopathic physician and herbalist. He is the best student of his mentor, the well-known herbalist, Dr. John Christopher. Schultze has the incredible temerity (and courage) to speak out about the harm pharmaceutical medicine has done to the health of America, and he reminds us that colon cancer is on the rise, as we continue to eat pathetically processed foods that are devoid of healing nutrients.

A FIRST STEP TO HEALTH

Health starts with the gastrointestinal tract: much of our immune power resides there, especially in the small intestines in the area known as Peyer's patches. When we consistently put dead, lifeless, filled-with-toxins food into our bodies, such as those found in our fast-food restaurants, the poor overworked liver, which is the master organ for detoxification, has to work overtime breaking down all these toxins instead of destroying cancer cells, which is one of its main functions.

One critic whom I know debunks the idea that health starts in the colon. He claims to have attended many autopsies that show no validity to the idea that layers and layers of toxic sludge inhabit our intestines. And yet my colon hydrotherapist, Annette Bray, R.N., has shown me the numerous parasites, mostly old and thankfully deceased, that are continuing to surface after several years of regular therapy. During autopsy, or colonoscopy, for that matter, when one views the inner aspect of the tubular colon with a fiberoptic light, the layers and layers of mucus cover over a sludge, giving the healthy pink appearance. This deception then gives us a false sense of comfort that all is well with the colon: we don't realize that all the toxic products residing there are prohibiting the necessary exchange of nutrients and waste that should be occurring. And we wonder why we are so sick with cancer, immune disorders, cardiovascular and neurological maladies.

IT'S SO SIMPLE

What is the answer? Start with water. We are comprised of 75 percent water, yet we constantly dehydrate ourselves with America's god: coffee and related stimulants. Coffee, tea, soda, and all of its variations, such as chai, cappuccino, iced tea with ginseng, dehydrate us and further keep us from healthy bowel movements. Every metabolic function in our body takes place in solution. To be really healthy we should be drinking one half ounce of water for every pound we weigh: between two and four quarts daily.

"How can I do that?" you ask. "I am a school teacher and I can only leave my room between classes." Well, folks, bowel and bladder health are vital. It is not to ignore the call for a bowel movement simply because we fear that the disruptive classroom forces will overpower the wallflowers in our absence. I suggest that we hire volunteers from our delightfully swelling force of seniors to travel from classroom to classroom every two hours to provide relief for those full-bladdered, stopped-up-coloned teachers. I even sent a letter suggesting such an approach to a high school principal on behalf of one of my patients. Just think about the pleasure of a glass of water not being such a terrifying concept!

And for those of you who dread using public toilets: get over it! How did we get so Victorian in our behaviors, when, on the other hand, we are so loose with our sexual behavior? Why worry about those sonorous farts we make when passing stool? After all, someone else is in the next stall doing the same normal thing.

My dear deceased husband, Paul, used to chant, "Wherever ye be, let thy wind blow free, for the want of air is the death of me." We have to get over the inhibitions we feel for natural body functions. They are keeping us unhealthy.

When drinking water, try it hot. Why we in America think that iced water is healthy for us is beyond me. It causes bloating, brings up gastric acidity, and chills us to the bone. As an herbalist having learned the teachings of traditional Chinese medicine (TCM), it is the kidney, rather than the liver, which is considered the master organ, and it hates the cold. Even the English drink their stout at room temperature. If you need a flavor, try a splash of lemon, which is also healing for the liver, and paradoxically alkalinizes the ph rather than acidifying it. Alkaline is the health promoting ph. And sip it throughout the day instead of dutifully chugging down your eight glasses iced cold and disrupting digestion.

BEYOND WATER

The next order of business for maintaining healthy intestines is putting more fiber in our diets. This does not include Twinkies, chocolate chip cookies and chocolate pecan turtles. Now don't get me wrong: I love Twinkies, chocolate chip cookies and especially dark chocolate pecan turtles and regularly give myself permission to partake; however, I do so only after I have given my body what it needs. My real favorite, though, is dark organic chocolate with coffee beans or hazelnut and toffee. They benefit endangered animals, making them environmentally inviting (brand: Endangered Species Chocolate).

And here's a healthy start for the delicate intestinal system.

Start the day with a delicious bowl of oatmeal and sprinkle ground flax seeds, raisins, and pumpkin or sunflower seeds over it, along with your favorite milk. I prefer a mix of rice and soymilk, and more recently, I found vanilla hemp milk (yummy), and of course, raw light or heavy cream, or cream fraische.

The flax seeds (easily ground in a small coffee grinder) are rich in *lignans*, which help to bind the excess estrogen produced by our bodies or introduced by animal protein sources that are tainted with it. If you loathe oatmeal, try bran flakes, or any of the other whole grain cereals. They are good substitutes, but eat them without the added sugar, please. Sugar serves to lower our very immune systems that fight off disease. Instead, add your favorite fruit in season:

banana, dried cranberries, blueberries, blackberries, strawberries. During the day remember to eat an apple and some grapes, figs, prunes or kiwi, strawberries, oranges, grapefruit, and melons, preferably those in season. Vegetables, legumes and whole grains should be the mainstay of our diets and can become tasty preparations with some very simple meal planning.

A LITTLE HELP NOW AND THEN

When occasionally we might need a laxative, the most harmonious use of these are the bulk laxatives containing psyllium. Better known as Metamucil or Citrucel or Konstyl, they are found in most supermarkets. Herbs with licorice and butternut bark can also be helpful. As the good doctor I am, I should warn you that licorice in excess can cause hypertension and a drop in potassium levels, but taken in sensible moderation, as suggested on packaging, there are usually no side effects. Herbal laxatives containing senna and cascara are more aggressive and might invite addiction to them, but in my mind a slight reliance is better than the alternative of constipation.

The Ayurvedic herb, triphala (contains amalaki, bibhitaki, and haritaki fruits) can help and is also very healthy. And what I am pleased to say about magnesium: it is heart, bone, sleep-inducing, as well as bowel friendly. Natural Calm Magnesium Powder is one of my favorites to stir into water before bedtime.

Lastly, if you take enough vitamin C, you will poop. Linus Pauling, discovering use of this important vitamin, used as much as forty thousand milligrams daily. It is a great aid to the immune system and it is heart healthy as well. I prefer Ester C because it is a buffered powder and can be stirred into juice or water. Be sure not to take chewable vitamin C: It can erode your tooth enamel if used regularly.

HOP TO IT

The next order of business is exercise. Now, don't let this thought evoke terror in your heart, as you envision yourself in a body-hugging body suit, pumping iron with Jane Fonda. Simply, walk. Lift some weights even if they are Campbell soup cans, while watching the tube after hours. Our bodies were made to move and that means more than passing from the refrigerator to the channel changer. Many of my patients are starting to work with private trainers at home, in privacy, and are discovering the joy of reducing visible cellulite along with feeling a whole lot better.

When we incorporate appropriate foods and exercise into our lives, our magnificent bodies respond and suddenly gerbil food pellet poop converts to healthy stools, and then our energy levels rise and depression lifts. Sounds too simple, doesn't it? But as with all things in this wondrous life, the *KISS* theory applies: keep it simple, smartgirl! For you see, when we have a *purposeful intention* to do something good for ourselves, our soul shines with the knowledge that we truly love ourselves. That is the key. I emphasize: you are important and deserve to feel good. Putting others' needs before your own is deadly and is a denial of God's great teaching: love thy neighbor as thyself.

Take Home Pearls

✧ Constipation kills and worsens brain fog, breast and ovarian cysts, uterine fibroids, and increases the risk of cancer.

✧ Fiber, water, and exercise aid healthy bowel movements.

✧ Ground flaxseeds, prunes, apples, are healthy, delicious, and promote elimination.

✧ Herbal laxatives (senna, cascara, butternut bark, licorice) are okay occasionally.

✧ Enough Vitamin C will make help bowel movements, as well as building our immunity.

✧ Magnesium is very heart and bone healthy and can promote healthy bms; great for sleep as well (my favorite: natural calm magnesium powder).

✧ Self love, taking our needs *first*, is key!

CHAPTER 11

Move Those Buns

You have to stay in shape.
My grandmother, she started walking five miles a day
when she was sixty.
She's ninety-seven today and
we don't know where the hell she is.
—Ellen Degeneres

Today in our high-tech world of medicine, all hospital rooms are complete with oxygen outlets for respiratory treatments. Not so in my days as a student nurse. Large, heavy, and difficult to maneuver tanks of oxygen lined the walls of the utility room. When a patient needed oxygen, we, the jack-of-all-trades nursing students, ran for a large cylinder, thank God on wheels, and hastened to the bedside of the needy recipient. It was not all that easy, however, because if that particular tank had not been "cracked" yet, we had to wield a wrench to open the outflow valve. One time, one of my hapless classmates happened to get a tank that had a defective off-on valve, and when she cracked open the master valve, so much pressure had developed that this several hundred pound missile careened out through the wall with the force of a canon!

My own memorable oxygen story unfolded one evening when, as a second year nursing student, I had charge of a sixty-bed ward with some very ill patients, many of whom required oxygen tents, which are rarely used today except perhaps on the pediatric unit to relieve a wee one with croup. At any rate, a red-haired young man with porcelain skin was inside of one of these tents, the plastic bubble covering the upper part of his body, then connecting to the tank. My evening had been particularly stressful with many new admissions to see to and dozens of intravenous bottles to keep a watchful eye on for resetting. As I rounded a corner to answer a patient's call-bell, I happened to see an oxygen tent completely fogged and heard the muffled cough of my redheaded patient. I glanced quickly at the oxygen gauge, and, to my horror, I saw it on Empty! I tore the plastic cover off the sweating, panting, suffocating man. Had that call-bell not been rung, my patient would have passed on to another plane, and I would have been up on manslaughter changes! In retrospect, I believe there are no coincidences; God was truly watching out for me.

The sixties were an exciting time for medicine, with new medical techniques and promising, sophisticated machines coming on line. But, in a way we lived in a time warp, where knowledge gleaned just a few weeks into the future might have saved someone's life if learned earlier. One of my more haunting experiences involved an elderly couple. The man had brought his wife into the hospital emergency room. She was gasping for breath, her lungs obviously filled with fluid, and suffering heart failure. After treatment, the woman apparently stabilized and was transferred to the medical ward on which I was working. After a couple of hours, this gentle, quiet man ran excitedly toward me, hastening me to come help his wife. She had stopped breathing. When I put my stethoscope to her frail chest, I heard no heart beat. Dear God, what was I to do? I had no idea.

My patient died, and the emotional impact of watching her grief-stricken husband walk slowly out of the hospital, stooped and bent, his felt hat in hand, hit me just two weeks later, as I was given instruction in the new cardiac massage procedure, which now is a well-known technique for reviving a stopped heart.

When I was just entering my teens, my friends and I would scale the fence into Palisades Amusement Park in New Jersey to avoid the thirty-five cent admission charge. I was always the last one over, getting my pants hooked on a spike. I would hear myself calling to my friends, "Hey guys, wait for me." I was known as a klutz.

I never really exercised; it was not part of my data bank. Rather, I was a hot shot, driving my fifty-two Chevy convertible, lovingly nicknamed "Bucky Beaver" because I bucked it all through second gear, all over town.

When I was in nursing school in 1961 my friend, Ginny, and I once sneaked onto private property owned by some folks who wrote horror stories. We were attacked by a couple of their vicious Dobermans and had to race back to the car at a speed that, because of my racing heart, let me know straight away that I was in far from pique physical condition.

When I was a nurse during the same period, the sixties, many physicians smoked, and they smoked blatantly in their offices, often when a patient was present. I remember one corpulent (that is a kinder word for fat) cardiologist who was so out of shape that he huffed and puffed just walking from his office to the reception desk! He always had a stogie, those aromatic Italian cigars which left me gasping after sharing close confines with him, like the elevator! What a role model for his patients! I used to just roll my eyes.

Now let's move ahead a couple of decades and flash onto the

sunny California scene, where thin, tanned bodies abound and folks jog, cycle, roller blade, and walk their dogs. There they eat a lot of sprouts and tofu and fat-free everything; they wouldn't think of consuming anything with a face, even fish or organic poultry.

Somewhere between these extremes is reality for most of us: I like to call it *balance.* And that is certainly necessary when it comes to exercise. How many of you can relate to the overzealous decision to start a new life: you go out and buy all kinds of fancy equipment, and of course, the svelte exercise clothing to prove you are a savvy consumer. You take to the streets or to the gym or to your basement, resolved to become trim and graceful. You probably overdo it and after three days every muscle you didn't know you had is screaming in pain. Little by little, your enthusiasm wanes, as you see that the scale is not moving downward, and perhaps even taking an upward slide. The next thing you know that wonderful treadmill or bike is serving as a tie rack, and perhaps it is even moving back into the garage where you know you will never go.

It was only as I began medical school in Mexico that I realized that some form of exercise would be essential to get me through endless hours of study.

So I began walking. Each night after a light evening meal, I would set out. One evening under a full moon, I bent down to tie the laces on my sneakers, when suddenly, I got nudged in the rear. Ready to stand and defend my honor, I whipped around, fists raised. For all my expectations, I was rewarded with the sight of a sleepy cow, greeting me with a gentle *moo.*

The most physically challenging period I ever experienced was later during my residency. The schedule was a grueling thirty-six hours on, twelve hours off for much of the week. Those hours on were mostly spent in the emergency room, assessing every sort of female abnormality possible, from overzealous menstrual cycles to ectopic pregnancies.

When my shift ended and I could look forward to a drive home for a longed for few hours of rest, I would inevitably find my car veering off to the gym where I withstood an intense, hour-long aerobics class. I so often felt reluctant to make this stop that I was surprised I actually did it; however, the commitment turned out to be a godsend. The exercise gave me more energy: I could turn my attention to my books for a while in study, then look forward to sleeping soundly for the rest of the night.

Moving your buns is essential. God gave us all these moving parts to use! There are many exercise experts out there who are happy to instill fear about getting fat and fill you with fatigue about what it takes to strengthen your muscular physique. But the truly important thing here is that you honor yourself by *exercising*.

I am not interested in hearing your sad tale of woe about your workweek and otherwise busy schedule. Who cares? Even bag ladies are busy these days. *Busy* is no longer an acceptable excuse to avoid exercise.

What is important here is that you *love and nurture* yourself by regularly setting aside some time for movement. Waiting until you get home from work is a sure way to fail: who isn't on vapors after a stressful day in the shop, at the office, in the classroom or at the computer. The secret, my gentle readers, is to get your bodies out of bed fifteen to twenty minutes earlier and walk, or lift weights, do yoga postures, row, or swim, or boogie to an oldies' tape. It doesn't matter what you do; just do something.

Exercise physiologists are starting to discover that it is not the rigorous nature of the exercise you do but the *regularity* with which you perform it. A good workout can be simply walking, but remember to get your heart rate up by at least twenty to thirty beats above your normal rate. The faster it resumes your resting rate after finishing exercise, the more fit you are. Don't go like gangbusters. For those of you who have been couch potatoes all your life, start five minutes a day, work up to eight minutes, then twelve, then fifteen. Progress until you are doing some form of aerobic movement, at least thirty to forty-five minutes three times a week. Aerobic activity includes walking, cycling, swimming and stair climbing. And be sure to warm up and follow with some stretching or yoga.

Remember, too the importance of *intention* as you approach and maintain your exercise program. When it is with an attitude of good will toward yourself, you are saying, "I count, and this is important to my health and well being."

During the darkest days of my depression, the only reprieve I got from my black abyss was the three days a week I pulled myself from the fetal position to attend my exercise class. *Always,* the darkness lifted, if for only a short time. Remember that exercise releases our bodies' own morphine bubbles, called endorphins, and they make us feel a whole lot better. What a boon for stiff, painful joints!

I encourage women with breast problems to swim: this enhances good lymphatic circulation, as the lymph is the fluid that removes all the toxins and cancer cells from our bodies. Rebounding on a small rebounder is an excellent way to move that lymph fluid.

I would like to mention my friend and associate in Women Wisdom and Wellness (WOW), Tahya, who teaches belly dancing to women with breast cancer, which is wonderful for their self esteem. She has been a musician and has taught the ancient arts of Middle Eastern culture for more than thirty years, and is a true dance diva.

Some menopausal patients of mine who have lost husbands tell me that it was only their commitment to "walk" every day that got them through their grief.

It is very important to remember contingencies: if you suddenly find yourself joyously walking outside daily in the balmy air, remember that it will rain or snow or sleet, so put Plan B into effect, so that you don't revert to couch potato status during the winter months.

If you exercise by yourself, you don't have to be all by yourself. Get some headphones and play a beautiful symphony or listen to my own personal favorite, the inspirational teacher, Deepak Chopra, or put on some affirmations by Louise Hay. As I sit on the rowing machine, I often find myself reciting the mantra, *God is my Source* or *Be here now,* or *how may I serve?*

Whatever you choose to do, do it with passion, vigor and resolve. I am disheartened and sometimes amazed to see how many women with great intentions start some form of movement but soon give it up because someone else's needs supersede their own. Who else in our lives is more important than we are?

Before the age of high tech, people always exercised and ate healthy. Heart disease and osteoporosis were little known entities. So, exercise! And do it because you deserve it. Your body knows when you are doing something good for yourself, and it will continue to work well for you for many, many years to come.

When we finally get it that God is not some judgmental guy with a long beard just lying in wait for us to "do wrong," but is instead an energy of pure, unconditional, divine love that pulses through our being when we allow it in, we might also understand that loving and honoring ourselves is the highest expression of life, the greatest tribute to God, and an essential experience before we can truly tend to anyone else's needs.

Take Home Pearls

✧ Some form of movement is essential for health.

✧ Exercise prevents osteoporosis and stiff joints.

✧ It is a natural antidepressant.

✧ It reduces stress and makes our bodies trimmer.

✧ Self love, taking our needs *first*, is key!

CHAPTER 12

Sexuality 101

Nothing in life is to be feared.
It is only to be understood.
—Marie Curie

Back in the sixties we didn't use euphemisms like sanitation engineer: you were a garbage collector, period. Likewise, sexually transmitted disease (STD) clinics didn't exist: they were called what they were: syphilis and gonorrhea clinics. Chlamydia, an STD caused by the microorganism chlamydia, at that time had not come into our awareness, nor had the human papilloma virus (HPV), nor had herpes to the degree that we know it today as a genital disease ... nor had AIDS.

Nursing students, such as I, had daily ward duties; we also were assigned to administer large syringes full of thick procaine penicillin and streptomycin to the long lines of patients wearing the scarlet letter of sexually transmitted diseases.

One day, sitting in the long line of self-imposed sinners was a young woman, pregnant, I was to find out later, with twins. As she sat under the fancy script sign, "Syphilis and Gonorrhea Clinic," she must have mused about the musical sound of those words, for when this preteen child delivered twin girls, their basinets sported the names, SeePhyllis and GoNora.

All my buddies growing up in Union City, New Jersey, were either only children like me, or they came from a family of all girls. One day our curiosity about male genitals got the better of us, and we five went round to call on Victor.

We enclosed our poor, hapless neighbor in a circle under a porch surrounded by protective latticework and instructed, "Okay, Victor, drop your pants."

We examined Victor with clinical precision, intending only to see why boys have outer plumbing, while we girls find ours embedded deep within. We in no way intended to traumatize our young friend. And in the years that have passed since that fateful summer day when I was a mere five years of age, I have often prayed for release from my guilt for perpetrating a deed that may well have caused Victor years of therapy for what he might have perceived as sexual abuse.

THE BIG "O"

When I lecture, I often reference Margo Anand, who wrote *The Art of Sexual Ecstasy* in 1989, a book that sheds much light on the subject of orgasm, that much sought after, dreamed about, schemed for phenomenon that sadly about 20 percent of women have never experienced. The big "O" is the talk in women's gatherings, in locker rooms, and upon therapist's couches.

Do you want to know the truth about orgasm? Anand quotes Alan P. Brauer, M.D., and Donna J. Brauer: "The average orgasm is only ten seconds long. The average frequency of intercourse is once or twice a week. That's twenty seconds a week, about one-and-a-half minutes a month, about eighteen minutes a year. In fifty years, that's about fifteen hours. For fifteen hours of ecstasy we devote how many thousands and thousands of hours thinking about sex, worrying about sex, daydreaming about sex, wishing for sex, planning for sex?"

Wow! Gives one pause, doesn't it?

One of my patients confided to me that she and her husband had been married for twenty-seven years and he felt a failure because he was never able to give her a vaginal orgasm. I told my patient to go home and hug her husband and tell him there is *nothing* wrong with him: most women do not have vaginal orgasms. Lest you be suspicious and feel still that you are missing out when it comes to the obscure vaginal orgasm, let me set your mind at rest: in my years of clinical practice, I rarely meet a patient who says she experiences a vaginal orgasm unrelated to the clitoris. Much mystery surrounds this subject.

Ah, the elusive orgasm!

How many of us have faked it? We feel as if something is wrong with us because our stalwart lovers are ready to blast off within three minutes, while we are hungering for hours of foreplay? God in His/Her infinite wisdom gave the genders different prep times, as it were, in order that we might avoid settling for the quickie. You all know what I'm talking about: the slam-bam-thank you-ma'am kind of lovemaking that simply releases the pressure buildup. (And that's all right, sometimes.)

But what about the slow, lingering kind of sex, that allows for the true meaning of intimacy to unfold? Have you ever thought about what intimacy means. Breaking down the word gives us its definition: *see into me.*

SHAMEFUL SECRETS

So many of us have experienced some form of abuse, whether sexual, physical, or emotional, that it is difficult to trust and give ourselves completely to the act of lovemaking. It is customary for me to ask all my patients if they have ever experienced any type of abuse in their lives. I hear so many devastating answers: one woman told me that she hated her breasts and was having a difficult time experiencing sexual intimacy with her beloved husband. I learned from her that her brother and uncle years earlier had fondled her breasts, and her guilt and shame had kept her all these years victimized. Slowly, after working with a sensitive therapist, she is learning to forgive her brother and uncle and herself and is moving on to experiencing a much healthier and more joyful sex life with her mate.

This business about forgiveness of self is so crucial: we are often unable to forgive ourselves because we feel so unworthy and unclean. But happiness is an inside job, and we have to dig deep to find it.

I'M NOT PERFECT

Our inability to enjoy sex is also a by-product of our endless self-criticism. Just listen to our toxic internal dialogue: "I'm so fat." "Look at all this cellulite and my ugly spider veins. How can anyone find me attractive?"

Well, if we are to find any pleasure in life, sexual or otherwise, we are going to have to learn to love ourselves in the package that we presently inhabit, and, further, to magnify our great assets with continual nurturing and respect.

LIFE'S LITTLE SELF PLEASURES

Those of you who are recovering Catholics may, like myself, remember being told by the stern padre and the well-meaning but shortsighted sisters that if we dared to masturbate we would grow hair on our palms and go blind. Well, thanks to God's great wisdom, there are no blind, hairy-palmed souls dancing about our planet, that we know of.

The truth, my gentle readers, is that our loving God wants only our happiness and pleasure, so surely the joyless, unhealthy teachings emerging from the church's hierarchy do not originate in the spiritual realm.

We have grown up with narrow Victorian mores, where society judges all clandestine behaviors severely and is quick to instill guilt and shame to nearly all sexual behaviors, but particularly to masturbation.

Masturbation is a word that most of us cannot utter without turning crimson, and certainly not many physicians or therapists are going out on a limb to recommend it, even in this age where focus on sex and passion reach near obsessive proportions.

To be sure, much of our sadness and frustration could be alleviated with self-pleasure: pleasuring ourselves is a stress-buster, a release from the pent up frustrations of unrequited love. It's certainly a viable alternative to unhealthy, destructive relationships, which many of us have surrendered to for physical gratification.

Too many of us have said *yes* when *no* is so much more prudent in a time when there are three million unwanted pregnancies yearly and an epidemic of sexually transmitted diseases, not the least of which is AIDS.

Widowed men and women, not able or willing to seek out new partners, do not have to be cut off from their sexuality. In their own privacy they can pleasure themselves whenever they want. The same goes for those folks whose partners cannot perform because of decreased libido caused by illness and the side effects of certain drugs. Though some men can get beyond the penis/vagina connection and take advantage of the multiple other erogenous zones, many sadly close down and go into their cave.

THE SURPRISING GOOD OL' DAYS

I was perusing one of the regular newsletters I used to receive called *Sex Over Forty*, or as they discretely call it, *S/40*, when I came across a review for a book called *Technology of Orgasm, "Hysteria," the Vibrator, and Women's Sexual Satisfaction* by Rachel P. Maines. It is a fascinating study of women's sexuality at the turn of the twentieth century. And, by the way, there is a magnificent docudrama DVD called "Passion and Power" based on this best-selling book. Award-winning filmmakers, Wendy Slick and Emiko Omori, tell the amazing story of one simple invention, the vibrator, and its relationship to one complex human experience—the misunderstood female orgasm.

At that time in the early 1900s, women seeing doctors for vague symptoms of malaise were often diagnosed as having *neurasthenia* (neurotic disorder), or *hysteria*. And they were prescribed a medical treatment that would certainly raise eyebrows today: regular, long-term clitoral manipulation to relieve their symptoms. And who was to deliver this medical treatment? Why their male physicians, of course. The treatment was, of course, couched in medical terminology, for certainly masturbation at that time was (and in some circles, still is) considered sinful, unhealthy, destined to cause madness, and it certainly was unmentionable.

Ms. Maines describes how a long list of symptoms for non-orgasmic women, including insomnia, headaches, restlessness, mood swings, depression, confusion, weepiness, and excitability, were collectively or individually considered symptoms of hysteria or neurasthenia. Now wait a minute! Aren't these our very symptoms of menopause?

Ms. Maine goes on to say that when the treatment of manipulating women's genitals began taking too long, the physician "was relieved" to be able to prescribe a new medical device: an electric vibrator, which had been invented by an English physician early in the 1880's. Ms. Maines writes "massage to orgasm of female patients was a staple of medical practice among some (but certainly not all) Western physicians from the time of Hippocrates until the 1920s. Mechanizing this task significantly increased the number of patients a doctor could treat in a working day!"

MIDDLE-AGED MYSTIQUE

Many of my forty- and fifty-year-old patients lament that their sex drives are in the basement, that sex is about as exciting as brushing their teeth? Well, sex at this hallowed age is different. I liken it to a burning ember, rather than the barn blaze it was when we were teenagers. And we have so many more interruptions to our sexual yearnings now than we did then. When we were teens we had no careers, spouses, children, grandchildren, elderly, chronically-ill parents, none of these to give all our life force to. Today our minds are so congested with the preoccupations of being everything to everyone, we have no time to fantasize and plan marvelous sensual trysts with our lovers. And to top it all off, our hormones are playing havoc with our sensuality.

Okay, so now we need to take action and plan a strategy, really take the time to do it. How about meeting your mate at the door wrapped in saran and sporting a large red bow in a very discreet spot: that should get him or her cooking! Plan an overnight at a local bed and breakfast. Give the children and/or elderly parents away overnight to some trusted friend, then party with your mate. Plan a long, relaxing bath in a tub surrounded by candles and tantalizing aromatherapy in the water. Cook a favorite meal, have your special dessert and wine, unplug the phone (all the phones, including the cell), turn off the beeper, Blackberry, TV, and play some delightful sensual, soothing music. None of this has to cost much; it just takes some imagination and a conscious effort.

I will share with you my Valentine's Day story. A few years back I was on call with the residents, supervising the Labor and Delivery Suite and the Operating Room for emergency admissions. I devised an elaborate plan, and, fortunately, the evening was slow, so I was able to execute it.

Years back when I was still doing deliveries and surgery, my office was connected to the hospital, and I had prepared a special examining room to which I would lure my unsuspecting mate. When he arrived to have dinner with me, I bade him wait for a moment in my office. I then scurried in to the examining room to change into a very sexy red teddy that left little to the imagination. I decorated that room with candles, incense and red balloons, then added a tape of soft music. And on the floor from my office to the examining room I sprinkled a path of red hearts. I then summoned my guy to follow the hearts, the end of this trail leading straight into my arms. I'll not kid you here. A hospital examining room complete with stirrup setups is a most intriguing and creative place in which to make love.

So what am I saying? Use your imagination. The brain truly is the main organ of sexuality, and attitude is everything, as the saying goes. When our attitudes are out of whack, sex doesn't work. Neither plunging neckline, nor spiky heels, short skirts nor crotchless hose will help if we're not approaching our sexual selves with gusto and glee and intensity. Don't bother making love with your body if your mind is doing the wash or balancing the checkbook. *Be here now* is the mantra for those consciously journeying to know God. Put *be here now* in your life, particularly during sex.

Speaking of God, one of my favorite authors is Andrew Greeley, a Catholic priest and Professor of Sociology at the University of

Chicago. He wrote a must-read book called *Sexual Intimacy: Love and Play*. In it he states that when two people who love each other come together and play, God smiles.

Let us help God smile more.

ELDER LOVE AND LUST

I have a delightful seventy-eight-year-old patient who once told me, somewhat shyly, that she often wakes up with an orgasm. I can't help but think that while she is asleep and dreaming she is in some way accepting her own body and soul needs and is assuaging her loneliness.

But many seniors have much difficulty coming to terms with their continuing sexual needs. They tell me that they're made to feel foolish when they talk of their need to express their sensual feelings.

One of the saddest experiences I had relating to love and sexuality among seniors occurred years ago when, as a nursing student, I did a rotation at a nearby nursing home.

Two of the residents, both widowed patients, had met and fallen in love. Annie was eighty-four and Joseph was eighty-seven. They shyly asked the matron in charge if they could have a quiet room together where they could demonstrate their love for each other. The cruel matron, who must never have experienced the joy of lovemaking, viciously denied them, then separated them, forbidding each to see the other again. The heartbreaking end to this true tale is that first Joe died, and then Anna followed shortly after. A modern version of Romeo and Juliet. Yes, I know of broken hearts.

UNCOMMON SENSE FOR COMMON COMPLAINTS

One of the most common complaints about what interferes with sexual satisfaction is vaginal dryness. Don't feel inadequate if you are not moist and wet all the time. This condition is a result of hormone imbalance, and it can easily be remedied with some estrogen or progesterone cream, as well as with Vitamin E oil. You can find several good lubricants on the market, but do not use Vaseline: firstly, it is a coal tar product, harmful to the vaginal area, and secondly, it prevents vaginal secretions from releasing and can cause infections. One of my all time favorite lubricants is organic 'unrefined' coconut oil. Not only is it wonderful for oral sex as it smells and tastes yummy, but as well it contains lauric and caprylic acids to prevent yeast infections.

There are many lubricating preparations on the market. Look for one containing Vitamin E, aloe and healing herbs. Speaking of Vitamin E, to moisturize your vagina and keep it healthy, cut open a Vitamin E capsule, and squeeze the oil onto your finger and rub it into your vagina nightly. Also, don't forget the testosterone cream (Chapter 3). Apply it to the clitoris.

And for those of us who have partners without erect penises, let's be creative and use our hands and mouth to pleasure our mate. We have dozens of erogenous zones throughout our magnificent bodies from which to derive and give pleasure. There are so many ways other than simply the vagina-penis connection. Cuddling and exchanging the day's adventures can be a most sensual experience. Quite frankly, going at lovemaking to achieve mutual orgasm can be hard work, while snuggling and kissing can be wonderfully healing. And regarding limp penises: remember, gay women do not have penises and they do just fine. To maintain erections, men can use cockrings, safer and probably as effective as Viagra and Cialis without the chemicals.

It is no coincidence that women on their honeymoon are prone to urinary tract infections, the so-called *honeymoon cystitis*. In the woman, the urethra, or bladder neck, is but four centimeters long, approximately one-and-a-half inches. It sits nestled within the vagina. Normally, a multitude of bacteria live harmoniously within the vagina and lower intestinal tract, but with frequent, repeated intercourse, there is irritation, and we are much more susceptible to bladder infections. When we get them, we often experience burning, pain and frequency of urination.

In the past, it was commonplace, after treating the infection with antibiotics, to enter into prevention mode: after each episode of intercourse, a woman was instructed to take Macrodantin, a urinary specific antibiotic. Well, I started thinking long and hard about this classical dictum and came to the conclusion that if a woman were blessed to have intercourse daily, then she would be using antibiotics constantly. Not only is such treatment costly but it opens the door to pesky yeast infections. Even more worrisome is the hit antibiotics take on our immune systems: constantly taking antibiotics lowers the body's natural healing ability by suppressing fighter cells.

A much simpler and very effective approach is *cranberry concentrate capsules.* Taking them after intercourse, or three times daily at the first sign of a urinary tract infection, can ward off the need for potent antibiotics. And the capsules preclude the need for drinking large quantities of cranberry juice: while fruit sugar is better than refined sugar, still it is sugar, and too much puts an unnecessary strain on the pancreas. It's better that your liquid be pure water, to flush out bacteria from the kidneys; it's also helpful with the bowel *and* for the complexion.

Keeping physically fit is another component for great sex. Do you remember the Kegel exercises you were taught in preparation for childbearing? Well, start using them again: they are great for sex. To review, in order to know how to perform them, start and stop your urine stream as you are voiding. Then, driving to and from work, practice these *squeeze and release* exercises five minutes twice daily: that is a song and a half on the radio. To be sure you remember, place a "K" on your steering wheel. If anyone asks what that is for, tell him or her it means "kiss me!"

Whatever we want to call it, sex is a most powerful form of communication and intimacy.

Take Home Pearls

✧ We are never too old to enjoy sex: after all, we *are* kids in wrinkled clothes.

✧ We do not need to have intercourse to have great sex.

✧ Most women do not have vaginal orgasms.

✧ Foreplay is essential...........and fun!

✧ Make dates with your mate: after forty the brain is our greatest sex organ.

✧ Organic coconut oil is a great and delicious vaginal lubricant, and it prevents yeast infections.

✧ Kegel exercises keep our vaginas juicy.

✧ Prevent urine infections after sex with cranberry concentrate capsules.

✧ Self love, taking our needs *first*, is key!

Part III

Becoming Whole:

The Final Frontier

CHAPTER 13

The Dance of Depression

Freedom is the absolute lack of concern about yourself.
—Florinda Donner

After finishing a yearlong stint in general surgery, I was admitted into the Department of Obstetrics and Gynecology, where I loved the diversity. A second-year resident, I was working every other night on call. We came on duty at dawn and worked through the night, finishing, if we were lucky, at five in the evening the following day. Then home, to eat, study, and sleep, only to get up at five o'clock and start that thirty-six-hour stint all over again.

One night when I had been up for what seemed like forever, I finally got to sleep around three AM and was having a fitful dream that someone was strangling me, when the telephone rang: it was the ER nurse telling me that a rape victim had just arrived. "On my way," I replied.

This rape victim was unlike those I had seen before. She was a seventy-year-old woman who had been asleep in her waterfront home along the Hudson River, when a young man broke in to brutally attack and rob her. When I saw this bleeding, broken woman, I simply sat down on the examining stool and wept. My hands trembled, not just from sleep deprivation, but from a rage that built inside me, that one human being could so harm, degrade and humiliate another.

After performing the necessary evaluation to satisfy legal evidence requirements for my inevitable trip to a court hearing, I left, still shaking, to return to my bed for an hour of sleep before morning report at six thirty. When I arrived for duty, a bit late, my attending physician, having heard about my trauma, chided me, "Can't take it, huh?"

I sincerely hope that I will never be a cold observer of life's inequities. But tending to the wounds of this tattered woman reminded me that each one of us suffers in some way. This episode was to be a prologue for my own wounds that I would soon be licking.

The hell of depression is a place I will never again allow myself to visit. It was on Mother's Day 1990 that I chose to end my life. No one who knew me would ever have believed it. I was the manic-depressive who never depressed. My norm was a high to others. I always had a sensational tale to tell and exciting webs of my perpetual adventures to spin. How could I, always the one with enthusiasm and encouragement for others, lose my will to live?

But you see, each day, as I showed the world my smile, my soul was screaming in agony, for I was living a life not of my choosing. In an effort to be the good girl and dutiful wife, I let my husband—this was number three—decide what was "best" for me, and he saw to it that my life was in his full control. Every night I was propped up against the big, puffy pillows in our huge bed, to watch a television program selected by him, my good husband, for my enjoyment.

I love books and music and playing with friends. These were the joys I relinquished when I chose to be with a sad, joyless man, whose lack of self-esteem enabled him to want to run my life. When I would bounce gaily home in my gym clothes, reporting on how a patient in the labor suite was progressing, he would glare at me, "You went to see your patient dressed like that?"

My young son even tried to warn me off this guy by telling me that this man was not right all the time and that my opinion counted, but I blew him off.

Where did that ballsy, independent, free-spirited lion lady go anyway? The one who had lifted me to such great heights and allowed me to achieve the unachievable!

I had sold out. I allowed my own hopes and dreams to die in the ill-fated attempt to please someone else.

It never works to do that.

When we do not stay in integrity, when we allow our soul's longings to be squelched, some part of us dies. It can be cell tissue, and we develop cancer or another deadly illness; or it can be, as in my case, the death of my soul, which carried with it a far more virulent, and possibly fatal, outcome.

My beloved God was not ready to let me off so easily, and my graphic attempt at swallowing one hundred sleeping pills and twenty-seven Valiums was thwarted by my guardian angel. Hospitalized and intubated, I remember awakening three days later to a woman psychiatrist peering into my tortured face, asking, "How do you feel?"

To which I would have shouted out, had I been able to speak through the tube dangling down my throat: "What the hell am I doing here? I should be singing with the angels about now."

The hand of God has always tweaked me, and this time was no exception. Struggling out from the depths of this nightmare, I mobilized myself with profound, healing anger and rallied to free myself from the bondage to which I had so willingly conspired.

Then a great truth came to me as if by a thunderbolt: your soul cannot be screaming *no* while your happy face is smiling *yes*. The schism of mind and soul is a deadly dance: there must be harmony and confluence if we are to have perfect health.

Empowering myself with a divorce that he initially requested, but which I orchestrated, I began the long climb home to health, to wholeness and to joy. I bought a condo, moved in with my two cats, and found solace and contentment for the first time in many years. My devastating suicide attempt was but a germinal seed onto a stage in my life where I was to find myself a true healer, (by my confession) credentialed and ready to recognize your pain.

Most of us have suffered depression at one time or another, often with good cause: the death of a mate, child or beloved parent is a traumatic life event that heals with the passage of time. But depression that comes from a failure to know our own personal power and speak our soul's truth is a different matter. This kind of depression is subtler, sometimes to a point we scarcely know it exists. But the effects are potent. We who live in the western world have a pattern of seeking help from someone else whenever we have a problem. Where our health is concerned, we go to the authority figure, the great white physician, and sometimes we aren't even satisfied with that. We further hone our requirements until we reach the specialist: a psychiatrist for our emotional ills, the gynecologist for our female complaints, the internist for our stomach problems. And we leave the soul's quest for the clergy.

But while we are compartmentalizing all our needs, we fail to realize one huge truth: no matter what our problems are, they are all connected. Always. No exceptions. So, it's no wonder we sink in to the depths of despair and depression, with feelings of helplessness and hopelessness when we don't feel well, because we have truly little chance for healing. Instead of tapping into our own soul energy, our *being* natures, we're too busy *doing* anything we can, hopping around hither and yon, to make the problem go away.

In many other cultures, the body-mind-spirit connection is honored, and true healing addresses every area of discord at once. Western medicine, on the other hand, is band-aid therapy at best.

Now don't get me wrong. There is no substitute for our wondrous medical intelligence on some matters. I would be the first to race to any hospital ER for my gunshot wound, my acute cerebral hemorrhage or auto accident. But for most other areas of illness, I would seek out a naturopathic healer with knowledge of herbs, nutrients, homeopathy, chiropractic and acupuncture. She or he won't interrupt me as I tell my story, as conventional physicians are known to do. (It is said that it takes a physician only twenty-two seconds to interrupt a patient trying to explain what's wrong!) The naturopath won't glance at the clock to see if we're overrunning the allotted fifteen minutes now set down by our HMOs. (And I haven't even asked my questions yet.)

There was a time in America when all healers were created equal, when they were permitted to care for their patients as they saw fit: allopathic medical doctors (M.D.s), doctors of osteopathy, herbalists, naturopaths, chiropractors, homeopaths and acupuncturists indeed were of the same echelon. Then the infamous Flexner Report of 1913 changed all that. That report, which came to be accepted as fundamental guidelines for a good medical education, placed scientific research and reliance on high technology as the prime focus in medicine, thereby all but destroying the holistic approach to healing and, further, ensuring an expensive brand of medicine. From that time forward only the allopaths and the pharmaceutical industry were honored as healers in this land, and we sadly witnessed the beginning of our healing decline and also our own personal loss of power.

Having gone through my adventure has given me a great edge on knowing you. It is no accident that at one time I invited all my new patients into my office, fully clothed, with the door closed so that I could touch them, soul to soul. My questions about one's physical history take very little time: that is the least challenging aspect of the meeting, for I have come to a sense of knowing that *all* physical symptoms are manifestations of our inner world.

When I first meet you I can see that your smile may be only pretense. What I really want to know is how you feel about yourself and your relationships with others in your life. I can start with the handshake. If it is limp and polite, and you speak to me softly and timidly and you cast your eyes downward and not directly at mine, I have immediate insight into your self-esteem. Body language is so telling: sitting with your arms crossed clues me in to knowing that you might be uncomfortable receiving information requesting a change in your thinking. Nails bitten to the quick tip me as to your sense of discomfort with yourself and your place in the world.

A classic example of how we patients are so intimidated by the authoritative physician showed up in my early days as an RN. I was working in a New Jersey community hospital and caring for a lovely patient called Mary. Her surgeon, a pleasant, competent southern gentleman, was a man of few words. We lovingly named him *Beep-Beep* after the roadrunner, because one moment he was there, and in the next he was long gone.

Mary had several concerns and questions about her surgery that would take place that day. I knew she wanted answers, but I also knew that *Beep-Beep* was going to be hard to pin down. I decided to try something different. "Write down all your questions," I advised Mary. "I will make sure you get your answers."

Mary did as I requested and when *Beep-Beep* entered the room, I ran to bar the door with my body and invited him to sit down. He raised his eyebrows but complied, actually sitting, and as Mary went through her list of questions, despite her fear and reticence, he actually gave her his time and attention. And he enjoyed it! We all felt empowered and fully honored by this full exchange. But why did it have to take a human barricade to get this job done?

Just recently, June, a nurse, came to my lecture seeking alternative therapies for a problem she was having. She was experiencing severe bleeding, constant headaches and other symptoms caused by the birth control pills her physician had prescribed for her. During our conversation after the lecture I reminded her that I was not her physician and could not ethically tell her to change her therapy. However, I did suggest that she tell her doctor what she had told me, that she wanted to stop the pills and try natural progesterone for a time to see if it could help.

Do you know how June answered this suggestion? She said, "He'll just tell me that I have to stay on the pills, and I don't want to hurt his feelings by telling him no." Isn't it amazing how, even where our own health is at stake, we will ignore our own needs in order to please someone else.

Natural healing is returning, and with it a glimpse of sanity to the healing professions. But it is causing much consternation among my colleagues who hold on tenaciously to the old ways. They still, for example, advocate a one-road-only approach for treating cancer: cut it out and destroy it with chemicals or radiation. They refuse to give attention to how that treatment wipes out the immune system, refuse to acknowledge the profound importance of whole, organic, live foods, and think silly any need to cleanse and keep healthy the intestinal system. They do not want to be bothered by a patient's emotional needs, nor do they value "treatment" through prayer and meditation.

Thankfully, some conventional doctors are coming around; they're becoming, as I like to call myself, recovering physicians and are more comfortable with these ideas and more willing to incorporate herbalism and natural healing into their practices.

Happily, I can report that major medical centers—Columbia, NYC, Mayo Clinic, Jefferson, Philadelphia—to name a small few, are seeing the importance of the mind/body/spirit connection. Dr. Mimi Guarneri, a cardiologist and head of the Scripps Medical Center in California, is reminding us that heart attacks can be prevented when we remember that the heart is the organ of love, and that besides a healthy lifestyle, we must remember to love ourselves and heal our psychic wounds with forgiveness and compassion. Her book, *The Heart Speaks*, is a wonderful affirmation of our power. And as the Bard says. "Go to your bosom, knock there and ask your *heart* what it doth know." He did not say *brain*, but heart. St. Francis of Assisi called the brain "Satan's lawyer."

One organization that I believe can best serve physicians who are truly interested in healing their patients is the American Holistic Medical Association (AHMA). AHMA, home to such famous healers as Bernie Siegel, Chris Northrup, Gladys McGarey and Patch Adams, is becoming a respected beacon, helping the physician to "heal thyself" before taking on the patient. AHMA is assisting physicians to comfortably relate all healing to love.

I would like to make a *case for* a phenomenal antidote for both illness and depression: *laughter*. The magical healing capacities of laughter are related in the marvelous book by the late Norman Cousins, *Anatomy of an Illness*. Cousins was struck with a crippling disease and basically written off, told by the experts that his cherished, active life would be cut short as he became progressively paralyzed. Well, he refused to accept this dire prognosis. He read and informed himself on how to fight it, and finally developed a unique plan of action. He asked his physician to administer massive doses of Vitamin C—one thousand milligrams per hour intravenously—and requested some old movies, the hilarious *Laurel and Hardy* series, and *The Three Stooges*. There has been much credence given to the healing elements of laughter ever since, because Cousins' illness went into remission, and he went on to write several inspirational works on the power of our minds in the process of healing.

Laughter is so healing and so emotionally uplifting because it calls on the body's natural painkillers called endorphins. Cousins' physician was a courageous advocate for his patient. Sadly, not many doctors would put their reputations on the line and agree to such unorthodox therapy.

Treat yourself each morning to a few good belly laughs: do whatever you need to do to laugh. If you get into the habit of laughing, it will come more and more easily. Deep laughter also increases your lung capacity and your circulation. In addition, truly, what is more fun than laughter?

A delightful new patient came to me one day. Eleanor said she had been feeling poorly, and she asked me a question common from my patients in the forties and fifties," Is this menopause or am I depressed?"

To which I usually answer, "It is all of the above."

She shared a recent Aha! experience, a small but mighty revelation. Eleanor said, "I woke up one day and realized that I was not saying anything good about myself, neither was I doing much laughing."

Since we have focused in this chapter on the benefits of natural healing for both the body and the psyche, I would like to end by sharing two extra special techniques that further heal all aspects of our body-mind-spirit:

- Hydrotherapy. This is a simple, safe healing mechanism. Sound too simple merely to take a shower? Try alternating hot and cold water for two minutes each for a total of fifteen minutes, ending with cold water! Not for wimps but it will fill you with an effervescent feeling.

- Skin Brushing. After bath or shower, take a natural bristle brush and scrub your skin briskly, starting at the feet and moving all the way up your body. This technique aids the lymph system and moves blood back into the heart and lungs. While brushing, sing your affirmations. How about saying this to yourself: *I accept you, I appreciate you, I forgive you, and I love you, exactly as you are.*

Another concept that is helpful in dealing with depression is meditation (see Chapter 16). Meditation clears cobwebs and allows the serene messages of the cosmos to reach through to the inner being. It teaches by its very gentle stillness how to live *in the moment.* When we are truly living in the moment, we are fully present to all of life's opportunities, and depression, which is usually based in regrets of the past or in fear of the future, wanes.

Take Home Pearls

✧ One major reason for depression is that we give our power away to another.

✧ Exercise creates happy bubbles called endorphins which prevent depression.

✧ Until we honor the mind/body/spirit connection, we can never truly be healthy.

✧ Laughter, skin brushing, and hydrotherapy improve our mood.

✧ Self love, taking our needs *first*, is key!

CHAPTER 14

Tribute to Leon

It has been ten years since I wrote *Menopause: A Spiritual Renaissance* and having reread it multiple times over these years, I was struck suddenly one day by the fact that a person who was a great part of my life for almost twenty years was totally missing from this book. Perhaps it was because I held sadness, guilt, and remorse when I thought of him that I orchestrated this glaring omission. Perhaps, also, and a great Aha! for me, is that Leon was the only man in my life who did not abuse me in some way.

Self esteem and the absence thereof has been a haunting, taunting leprechaun that followed me through the many long dramas in my life's journey. And so, as I analyze my behavior, I realized recently that someone who loved me unconditionally for all my bitchiness and spoiled bratness could not fit into my dysfunctional belief system.

We met in Tampico, Mexico. His black hair and gentle blue eyes engaged me at once. An only child like me, he endured the traumas surrounding families who lost everyone but their nuclear family in the Holocaust. We met, learned to laugh and love, study together, and dine on the wonderful delights of Mexico.

Driving to and from Mexico afforded us many, many hours to share stories. He was horrified to hear about the many one night stands I pulled off during the sixties and seventies.

"How could you think so little of yourself that you allowed men to use you like that?!" he would ask, shocked at my offhanded comments.

Because Leon was an intellectual—and I mean that in the fullest sense of the word—studying the tenets of biochemistry, histology, and pathology bored him. And what's more, taking tests in Spanish was very difficult for him. So I tutored him through our studies. He had done cancer research in Jefferson University, Philadelphia, and in Dartmouth University in New Hampshire.

An amazing true story of his integrity for pure research placed him on an elevator at Dartmouth. It just so happened than a cage full of mice involved in a top-notch research project was being transported to another lab. On the same elevator, there was a cart full of water pitchers being delivered to a patient floor. Leon, tall, and with a great presence, was reading an important scientific paper, and accidentally, knocked one of the water pitchers over, on top of the cage full of mice. A fascinating thing began to happen: the color on the backs of the mice started washing off! My Leon was inadvertently responsible for revealing a terrible truth in the research world: the world-famous doctor responsible for this experiment had willfully painted the backs of these mice to prove an important finding in the cancer world, and Leon was the hero responsible for bringing this to light and sending this researcher into disgrace!

Eccentric was not a big enough word for him: he epitomized Thoreau's dictum of stepping to the beat of a different drummer. One summer, as we drove back from New York to Tampico, we stopped to visit my cousin, Rose, who was then living in New Orleans. Up at dawn, she found him reading his Bible. A devout and Orthodox Jew (and one who questioned *everyone*, and challenged the teaching, even of the Rebe), he never spoke of his dietary requirements. And as fate would have it, Rose, so proud of her cooking talents, served a luscious baked ham that night. He politely ate a piece, and said nothing. Keeping harmony and not humiliating his host was more important to him than his laws.

We fell in love and ultimately lived together in a hotel near our school. His old Dodge, which we called the Batmobile, took us everywhere, and when we took off on semester break to travel back to the northeast, his trusty car made it, despite breakdowns requiring mechanical skills which, among so many other things, Leon possessed.

Finally finished with our schooling and back in the states, Leon pursued a urology residency in Long Island and I a year of general surgery, then an OB-GYN residency in New Jersey.

Our lives were tortured by his mother's desire for him to marry a Jew. Yet, he loved me, and continued to love me through my next three marriages. When Paul, my second husband died, I embraced him back into my life. When my next husband entered my life, I said good-bye once again to Leon. After my second divorce, I again pursued him, but was mean and taunting because he was so busy in his residency that we could spend little time together.

Leon was a collector of things, many wonderful things: antique radios, spiritual volumes of Judaica, but as well newspapers, salt, pepper, napkins, and tea bags. Finally, saying good-bye to him for the last time in 1993 with my final marriage, I did not see or speak to him until 2006 when a thought of him came very strongly to me.

There is no mistake: I had some major karmic debt to repay this man for all the hurt I had inflicted upon him. He loved me for all time, never marrying. I listened—as we must—to my intuition—and reached out for him. Saddened profoundly by what followed, I found him, very ill, suffering the ravages of diabetes, kidney failure, hypertension, and an amputation from a life-threatening bone infection.

Tragically, he owned a large, very expensive home in New York State; no longer able to work, his debts were mounting. With my hopelessly optimistic Mary Poppins attitude, I was certain that I could assist in his healing. I brought Leon to my home, began installing many of his belongings, and helped him as much as I could to pay his bills. With a determination I persisted, even though I was losing my soul—once again.

Many other bleak events were catapulting me into despair. My esteemed father, at eight months short of his one-hundredth birthday, died. My beloved cat, Shadow, on the cover of the original edition of this book, died, and I felt my internal pilot light on flicker.

Caring for this man was a full time job. Often in the middle of the night, as he was sliding into diabetic insulin shock, I would bolt to the kitchen to prepare a sugary drink to save him from unconsciousness. A labile diabetic, finding blood sugars surging dangerously upward, I would prepare his insulin with shaking fingers. It had been long ago that I ran an emergency room. And taking care of patients was a great deal different from caring for a loved one.

There is so much more to say, but I came full circle to realize my repetitive need to care for men and change myself to make them love me. Leon did in fact try to inflict the guilt of his illness upon me, inferring that if I had not abandoned him, he would not be ill. And for a time, I accepted this guilt, even though I teach that guilt accomplishes nothing and should never be part of our belief systems.

The fun-loving, carefree life we had together in Mexico was gone, to my sorrow.

I had a take on these illnesses of his. I felt that with his undying dedication to his patients, Leon worked himself into the disease which would ultimately kill him. The unhealing fracture of his heel that led to his amputation was a direct result of his dedication to his job and his patients: giving and giving and giving to them and not to himself. Is this starting to sound familiar?

The little 'blip' on the cardiogram interpreted by an intern catapulted him into an unnecessary cardiac catheterization, the dye of which destroyed his already frail kidneys damaged by years of uncontrolled diabetes. What does the metaphysical world say about diabetes mellitus? "Lacking sweetness in life." And speaking of kidneys: he was on the list for a donor. As fate would have it: *I was a perfect match*!

I was about to give a dying man with a pathological need to hoard everything he ever acquired, one of my kidneys, as if I were bringing a gift to a birthday party. Now, remember, this was all of 2006, when I thought I had finally shucked off the need to give myself away to everyone else, without establishing boundaries and or considering my own needs.

I also recall that I was about to convert to Judaism to please his mother. I took Hebrew lessons and immersed myself into the teachings of the Old Testament. All of this was noble, but it was at a time in my life where my chameleon status of changing to make everyone else love me was a constant companion to me. As well, my reverence for the large tomes of medical knowledge, so prized by Leon, kept me in that place of obeisance and dutiful, unquestioning respect for our hallowed profession.

Struggling out of the confused dedication to Leon's tenacious hold onto religious and medical dogma, I began challenging his beliefs. And as sick as he was, he bellowed at me, accusing me of blasphemy when I read to him the Sufi poet, Hafiz's works, that spoke of the sensuality of God, and our oneness with God.

When I contested the absurd teachings of medicine, that everything is a deficiency of drugs—a headache is an aspirin deficiency, depression a Prozac deficiency, high cholesterol a Lipitor deficiency—he gave me the reams of research contesting my perspective, most of them, of course, provided by the pharmaceutical industry.

Something was not working here. I allowed my guilt to surface as he reminded me that he had loved me all these long years, never marrying. How could I continue to break his heart?

Needing to remove myself, I flew to California to the Chopra Center where I regularly studied with my beloved teacher. I made an appointment with David Simon, M.D., Deepak's partner. This Yoda-like man, sardonic and loving, wrapped in a piercing eye contact package, listened carefully to my story, as I admitted my great despair and fatigue.

He said the words that stung me like a hornet's hive: "Let me get this straight: you are a heroin addict, and you are getting ready for your final, terminal overdose!"

Had he pointed an uzi at me and pulled the trigger, the jolt could not have been more forceful: I was shocked into seeing the reality of my love addiction; in that, I was granted a reprieve from my need to fix everyone and be loved by everyone.

What do we say: we always teach that which we ourselves most need to learn? Leon's role in my life was to teach me two major revelations: we can and should love unconditionally and compassionately without the attempt to change another. Most importantly, if we love ourselves unconditionally and compassionately, we do not need to change ourselves for another to love us.

Take Home Pearls

✧ We always teach that which we need to learn.

✧ If we love ourselves unconditionally and compassionately, we do not need to change ourselves for another to love us.

✧ Guilt sucks: forgive your unhealthy thoughts and move forward!

✧ Self love, taking our needs *first*, is key!

CHAPTER 15

The Elusive Self-Esteem Gene

No one can make you feel inferior
without your consent.
—Eleanor Roosevelt

A prime responsibility for nursing students was to assist interns during
special procedures. One patient with meningitis was scheduled for a
spinal tap, a technique for removing spinal fluid from the lower back
through a needle stick. The intern was using Novocain to numb the
area where the needle would be inserted.

This intern, a tall, dark-haired Armenian chap, affable and
conscientious, asked me to gather the necessary equipment. I ran to
several different spots to retrieve the goods. For some quirky reason
the tiny glass ampoules of Novocain were sitting in a little plastic
container alongside a potent medication called Levophed, used when a
patient is in shock. Not only is this drug very concentrated, requiring
dilution before being administered intravenously, but there is a bold
warning on the drug insert page to prevent at all costs this medication
from entering the subcutaneous tissue beneath the surface of the skin,
because it could cause a profound decrease in blood supply to that
area, resulting in gangrene.

You guessed it: instead of grabbing the pain numbing Novocaine, I got the Levophed. Then ignoring Rule #1 to always check medications carefully before administering, we went ahead. As the doctor was injecting our unsuspecting patient, I remember him wincing and complaining of discomfort. Our poor patient was having a dangerous drug injected into the soft tissue of his back, and it wasn't until the tap was completed that I discovered my grievous error. I swooned in stark terror at my mistake. Pale and shaking, I slunk in to see the doctor and confess my deed. That handsome face became chalky white and little beads of sweat immediately broke out on his upper lip. He didn't yell at me, as certainly I deserved, but instructed me to keep watch on the patient throughout the night. We made out an "Incident Report," which is a medico-legal requirement, but didn't let our patient know about the mistake. How I agonized throughout that night and how I prayed to God to forgive me. Fortunately, this young man suffered no ill effects. You can imagine my profound relief and gratitude. What a way to learn a lesson!

The summer before I entered nursing school, I went to Cape Cod with some high school buddies. Staying in the Buccaneer Motel in Provincetown, Massachusetts, we met some lovely chaps from Pennsylvania. Herbert was my personal choice, and we maintained a correspondence by mail for six months at which time he invited me to a New Years Eve party in his hometown, Philly.

What follows is a glimpse into the emotional frailty and tottering self-esteem that I would carry with me for the next forty years.

In preparation for my momentous date with the desirable

Herbert, my mother had sewn me a magnificent dress: it was a jewel-green velvet skirted number topped with spaghetti-strapped mint-green brocade. It was gorgeous! And I was mightily excited.

I had always been blessed with creamy, flawless skin. But just days before New Year's Eve, I was graced with the appearance of twenty-one pimples on my face, one for each year I lived on the planet. Now I was devastated! But with the help of some makeup, I was able to cover it up successfully. I boarded a train in my green confection, and, if I do say so myself, looked fairly well turned out – beautiful, in fact. Herb greeted me at the train station with a look, I noted, of instant approval.

If it had been at all within my power, I would have pulled that night off with great success. But it seems that was not to be. My miserable self-esteem surfaced, and for what reason I can't even explain, I felt compelled to explain to each and everyone present that night the story of my pimple breakout. The entire evening, of course, was a disaster, irreparable, and I never heard from Herb again.

My self-esteem wouldn't improve much as time went on. Later, as a nurse when I was bound and determined to find "Mr. Right," longing for a "true love" relationship, I would sit with my best friend night after night in a restaurant near the hospital staring at various medical student possibilities, each one of whom I was convinced would become my soul mate. Most of these guys I had neither met nor even talked to, but still I fantasized about becoming involved in a meaningful, heart-stopping relationship. My continuing need to be known and loved would follow me through many years of searching, until finally one day I became enlightened to the knowledge that it was actually my own self—me—from whom I wanted to know love and acceptance.

THE IMPORTANCE OF SELF

I am constantly reminding my patients of one of the most important Commandments: *Love thy neighbor* as thyself. Why "to love thyself" is such a hard concept is beyond me, yet we have all bought into "do for others—first." We allow a most insidiously pathological emotion, *guilt*, to guide our actions. Societal pressures compound this. What we must press into our data banks is that *if we cannot love ourselves, we cannot love another. Period.* And what kind of role models are we for our children, when all they see is mom and dad on vapors as they fly about hither and yon performing every chore imaginable to prove what stellar parents we are. Certainly, it doesn't take a Rhodes scholar to deduce that our children might well decide that parenting is a drudgery-filled, dead-end job.

Our lives must start with ourselves. Anything given to another while our own needs remain unmet borders on martyrdom. A well-known practice on airplanes punctuates this fact and provides for us the perfect metaphor. What do airlines tell us about handling an oxygen emergency in flight? *Put your own mask on first.* Are you starting to get it?

Self-love includes the ultimate requirement for self-healing: *forgiveness.* Living with anger, vindictiveness and resentments serves no one. It's no surprise that those negative emotions don't ever nail their target: they make rapid u-turns and boomerang right back to us! A Chinese proverb reminds us that if are going to continue being angry and resentful, we'd better dig two graves!

Betty Eadie's, *Embraced by the Light,* speaks of a woman's near-death experience during which she meets up with God. Up to the time of this encounter, the woman has lived an ordinary life with ordinary experiences, just like the rest of us. She has also carried with her the baggage of guilt and resentment, just like the rest of us.

The message she receives from God and brings back with her for the rest of us is simple, yet profound: *Love yourself and all others unconditionally, and forgive yourself and all others* unconditionally.

On that fateful day at age eighteen when I went to my high school guidance counselor and asked, "What should I be?, nobody suggested that I could become an aeronautical engineer, lawyer, doctor, physicist or racecar driver. My options were only two: nurse or teacher

Being told that my gender allowed for so few career choices, however noble they may have been, in retrospect was a gift, because a germinal seed was planted, which would lead to a wonderful personal evolution. I would have stayed a nurse, but for the mass cultural mindset that demands that respect and attention be paid to the physician. Wanting that same respect and attention for myself pushed me toward attaining my M.D. degree. My self-esteem and self-assuredness, however, lagged miserably behind my goal setting. And the nursing environment from which I was emerging certainly was no help; the nursing structure never supported the idea that we nurses were anything more than second-class citizens. Even despite my long uphill climb to achieve what appeared to be an enviable position, I continued to feel inadequate, allowing the mean little voice inside to taunt me, reminding me how stupid and ill-prepared I was. During the darkest days of my depression, I remember lying in bed, sleepless, forcing myself to go through the steps of surgically performing a vaginal hysterectomy, a formidable task for me as this area of gynecological surgery was the one in which I was the most poorly taught. That little niggling ego continued its taunts and jeers at my inadequacy, wearing down my defenses, and more importantly, eroding the kernel of self-esteem that represented my identity to the world. As a result, every flaw, every weakness in my knowledge, I wore pathetically on my sleeve for the world to see and exploit.

We are all mirror images of each other, so that when I think that I am less than perfect, so also does every friend and stranger I meet. Many life events bring to the surface many of the insecurities, perceived "failings," and little secrets that we have tucked away into the farthest depths of our soul. For so long throughout our lives, we have ignored them, believing they might simply go away. But often later in life we are privileged to get to know these aspects of ourselves. Privileged, you ask? Yes, because they provide the keys to our true nature, from which satisfaction and fulfillment emerge.

The examining room is where I share what I call "sacred dialogue." My conversations with patients demand that I be present, truly present. And for that I must take care of myself first. Sometimes it isn't easy fitting in all the aspects of nurturing my physical, emotional, and spiritual requirements, but I make time anyway. And the first thing on my agenda, after feeding my magnificent cats, Karma, Dharma, Jewels, and Justin, is meditation. Without starting my day with deep breathing, prayer and an attitude of gratitude, all of which takes about twenty minutes, I can feel fragmented, scattered, and most importantly, not present. I must be *with you* to hear your story so that we can work together to mastermind a plan.

I am struck by how conditioned women are: the minute they enter my examining room, they get on the table, lie down, and spread their legs.

"Wait a minute," I say, "I want to look at all of you, not just your pelvis!"

Then I lighten them up with this scenario: "Imagine a CEO, well-dressed in an impeccably-cut Italian suit, entering an examining room. In walks a gorgeous female urologist. Without any further ado, the CEO unbuckles his trousers, drops his drawers, and bends over to receive his prostate check. Can you just imagine that?"

We laugh, and now you may be wondering what all this has to

do with self-esteem. Well, it's subtle, but think about it. We women have been allowing medical doctors to have their way with us, without their knowing or caring who we are. Not great for the self-esteem, eh? There is much more to you than your pelvis. Unfortunately, the super-specialists think that only "their part" counts.

When I consider the entire human being, I learn so much about her. Along with the "human connection" of actually looking an individual in the eye, I can tell much by simply scanning the outer body. For example, dry brittle hair might signal thyroid dysfunction or hormone imbalance or a lack of essential minerals and essential fatty acids; reddened eyes can hint at problems ranging from sleeplessness and anemia to poor-fitting contact lenses. I even diagnosed one woman as having AIDS because she exhibited a thrush on a throat exam (white spots caused by a fungus).

What is so pervasive in conversations with my fellow goddesses is their lack of self-acceptance, lack of self-esteem, lack of self-love. I usually begin these talks with the question, "Are you healthy?"

The answers I get back are mostly self-deprecating. "I'm healthy, but I'm fat." "I'm healthy, but I'm not exercising as I should." "I'm healthy, but I'm eating all the wrong things." Sometimes I feel as if I'm in a confessional complete with white collar, listening to the sinful unburden themselves. What I wouldn't give to hear one of you say, "I'm healthy, happy and satisfied with myself just as I am. I just want to make a few minor adjustments."

Louise Hay is a brilliant metaphysical lecturer and teacher, and I offer thanks to Jill Kramer at Hay House for letting me reprint this excerpt from Louise's book, *Gratitude: A Way of Life.*

I have noticed that the Universe loves gratitude. The more grateful you are, the more goodies you get. When I say 'goodies,' I don't mean only material things. I mean all the people, places and experiences that make life so wonderfully worth living. You know how great you feel when your life is filled with love and joy and health and creativity, and you get the green lights and the parking places. This is how our lives are meant to be lived. The Universe is a generous, abundant giver, and it likes to be appreciated.

Gratitude brings more to be grateful about. It increases your abundant life. Lack of gratitude or complaining, brings little to rejoice about. Complainers always find that they have little good in their life, or they do no enjoy what they do have. The Universe always gives us what we believe we deserve. Many of us have been raised to look at what we do not have and to feel only lack. We come from a belief in scarcity, and wonder why our lives are so empty. If we believe that "I don't have, and I won't be happy until I do..." then we are putting our lives on hold. What the Universe hears is: "I don't have, and I am not happy," and that is what you get more of.

When I awaken in the morning, the first thing I do before I even open my eyes is to thank my bed for a good night's sleep. I am grateful for the warmth and comfort it has given me. From the beginning, it is easy to think of many, many more things that I am grateful for. By the time I have gotten out of bed, I have probably expressed gratitude for eighty to one hundred people, places, things, and experiences in my life. This is a great way to start the day.

In the evening, just before sleep, I go through the day, blessing and being grateful for each experience. I also forgive myself if I feel that I made a mistake, or said something inappropriate, or made decisions that was not the best. This exercise fills me with warm fuzzies and I drift off to sleep like a happy baby.

We even want to be grateful for the lessons we have. Don't run from lessons: they are little packages of treasures that have been given to us. As we learn from them, our lives change for the better. I now rejoice whenever I see another portion of the dark side of myself. I know that it means that I am ready to let go of something that has been hindering my life. I say, "thank you for showing me this, so I can heal it and move on." So whether the lesson is a "problem" that has *cropped up or an opportunity to see an old, negative pattern within us that it is time to let go of, rejoice!"*

There is so much wisdom in that passage: our thoughts *do* create our reality, so if we are always complaining about what we don't have instead of blessing what we do, we just keep ourselves in the mire of despair. That is why I stress over and over that we must love ourselves, as we are. We are all jewels in the making, works in progress. The phrase, *you can look at the glass as either half empty or half full*, may seem trite, but it is profound in its meaning.

Martyrdom is pathological and actually quite harmful to loved ones who might be receiving our constant care. When our children witness our harried demeanor and seething resentment about always being on call for them, they may well get the notion that motherhood stinks. Why not give your child the gift of witnessing you taking care of your needs. That implicitly gives *them* permission to nurture themselves, and the sick pathological cycle of martyrdom will at last be broken.

One of the most toxic attitudes we have originates inside our own heads. Have you ever gotten a compliment, then said, "Yeah, but ... " Patrick Collard is a master intuitive and body worker, who has developed a tape series called *Success Without Sabotage,* in which he speaks of our inability to love self by "yeah, butting" everything. We need simply say, *thank you*, and then give ourselves a hug.

We women have entertained for years images of ourselves as second-class citizens. After all, we just got the vote less than one hundred years ago. Women in certain third world countries still walk ten paces behind their men folk, and they cover their magnificent locks to the outside world. In certain countries male children are considered superior to female, and women are still aborting themselves if ultrasound reveals a female fetus in order to avoid losing their dowry or even their lives.

Even though we in America have legislated equality, we remain toxic in our thinking, buying in to all the teaching of our inferiority.

So my dear sisters, I want you to do special practice each and every day, four times. And practice this in front of a mirror as this is so much more powerful: Look yourselves in the eyes, the looking glass into the soul, and say out loud the following: *I (recite your name), I accept you, I appreciate you, I forgive you, and I love you, exactly as you are.*

Take Home Pearls

✧ Dry skin, brittle hair may signal thyroid dysfunction and essential fatty acid deficiency.

✧ Lack of compassion for self worsens our depression.

✧ Gratitude for all we have and for the good yet to come is essential.

✧ Self love, taking our needs *first*, is key!

Chapter 16

Opening the Soul –
The Hidden Cure

*The failure to cultivate virtue,
the failure to examine and analyze what I have learned,
the inability to move toward righteousness after
being shown the way,
the inability to correct my faults—
these are the causes of my grief.*
—Confucius

Danu came from Chicago. She was a pale-skinned, blue-eyed beauty with red hair the color of an autumn tree in its glory. She bubbled into my office for her annual "lube job" and our wonderful connection began. You know when that word "connection" has the meaning it is there to evoke: we had an instant rapport; whatever subject we touched, it seemed at some juncture our lives had been together.

To digress for a moment, my initial interview with patients used to be in my office, a comfortable, sacred space surrounded by my favorite books. They sat, along with a terrarium and desk plants, on a huge table I converted into an enviable desk. On the wall are pictures of nursing mothers, babies and many plaques espousing self-esteem and the power of womanhood.

My office was, in fact, the office library. When I joined the practice, there were no rooms at the inn for me, save this one. The senior partner said, "Helene, you can do anything at all with this room, but you cannot remove the board table." Well, initially my heart sank as I gazed at this 10-foot long oval table. But with a bit of creative planning it has become the most comfortable office I have ever inhabited. I include this rambling description because I have found over the years that when we put a patient clad only in those pathetic Johnny coats (at least ours are cloth) and sit her near-naked on a cold table replete with stirrups, it does not engender the kind of atmosphere where a woman can bare her soul (her body is enough!) to such intimate questions as have you ever been sexually or physically abused?, do you enjoy sex and do you regularly experience orgasms? and how do you deal with avoiding pregnancy during intercourse? and do you like your work?

I have named my desk the "crying" desk and am sure to always have a tissue box to offer my ladies, for invariably, my searing questions spin some buttons and they often weep uncontrollably. Ah, but what a wonderful first step to healing; catalyzing their entry into counseling where these traumas can be dealt with and often laid to rest through forgiveness work is one of my gifts.

Back to Danu: as we were getting ready to exit my office and enter the examining room, she casually asked a question that had the effect of a bomb dropping in my life. It would change my life inextricably and for all time. She said, "Oh, by the way, I teach meditation. Are you interested?"

To which I answered, "What's that?"

How many times can you see or hear something and it simply passes you by until, one day, you *get it?* I vaguely remember attending a meditation class in the sixties where a guru uttered strange syllables like "Ohm" and "shanti, shanti, shanti." Incense burned, and there were silk shantung wall hangings of strange gods and goddesses along with knowing initiates sitting cross-legged in what I now know to be lotus position. However, at that time, my life was frenetic, filled with frantic household and motherhood duties and nursing responsibilities. And my marriage hovered between terror-filled abusive episodes and soul-dragging banal communications. There not only was no time to go within myself, there also was no understanding that to do so would bring me any measure of peace, grace, tranquility or wisdom.

Until my fiftieth year, I had sought external solutions to all my queries into life. It was always someone else's wisdom, someone else's philosophy, and someone else's get rich quick scheme. It is often said, however, that when the student is ready, the teacher appears.

Then one day I heard Jesus' words for the first time: *better things than I you can do.* And the concept that God is within us, around us, actually everywhere, an idea so blasphemous to certain religious teachings, made the most amazing sense to me.

My meditation practices now take priority in my life. Twice daily for at least twenty minutes I go within, allowing the pressing stresses of the day to dissolve, as I permit thoughts to pass by without giving power to them. I concentrate on my breath, the life force without which we could not survive. (How many of us take the magic of our respiratory center for granted!) There are many techniques to meditation: concentrating on the breath, or a flame; mantras, sounds and syllables can give meaning and peace. It doesn't matter, really, about the technique: the importance is the essence of meditation, our relinquishing of the hustle and bustle of our lives, our scattered, often negative, chatter to indulge for a time in the still, quiet sound of silence.

"Be still and know that I am God" is an expression I love. I have been taught that God does not show up in windstorms, in floods or tornadoes, but in the utter whisper of a butterfly's flapping wings; in the faint breeze on a stagnant day; in the twinkling of a distant star. And God comes in the stillness of our meditation. It is said that prayer is talking to God, and that meditation is listening to God.

During this quiet repose we are able to tap in to the cosmic wisdom that has been available to us always. We have access to all the great sages, as well as the scoundrels, for the energy that is our essence can neither be created nor destroyed. Herman Melville of Moby Dick fame said, "Silence is the only voice of God."

This practice has become a springboard to bridge my spiritual life and my physical life, and each day, they become more and more one and the same.

The traditional paradigm for so many of us is to view God as a far away diety, to be visited on Saturday evening or Sunday morning when we pay homage with our prayers and hymns. I cannot help but view most religions as pompous and arrogant, because instead of uniting humanity, they separate us, each one espousing that its way is best. "My God is better than your God, and surely you will not enter the kingdom of heaven if you don't come through my set of gates." This belief system has been the underpinning for all the religious wars, world wars, bigotry and a multiclass system whose preachings promote the concept that "I am in charge, you are my followers."

Religiosity, as interpreted by man, separates. Spirituality, on the other hand, unites us all to realize that if God is present everywhere and contained in each one of us, then obviously no one man is any less or better than another.

I like to teach in my lectures that the first fifty years is dress rehearsal; the second fifty is real time!" For the first fifty, I definitely was asleep. My life was what happened around me and to me. I had little input and was not in charge. I always went outside myself for the answers.

My new teachers and mentors, however, helped me to see that living right now, in present time, is the only place to be. Indeed, it is the only reality there is. *Be here now, I like to say. L*iving in the dead past or the phantom future permits the entry of all those negative little voices calling forth fear, anger, rage, hate, vengeance, resentment, guilt, envy--all of the emotions that squeeze out love and forgiveness. When we relinquish the need to hold on to all these emotions, then we heal.

A great example of *not* being in the moment is in following to the letter and in order the items on your to-do list. When I used to do that, when I was on item number one, my mind was already catapulting ahead to number eight on the list, and I was fretting about how I could tackle it. Meantime, the present task was lost to me. One day, as I was *not* living in the moment, a funny and also not-so-funny thing happened: I was pulling into the hospital parking lot for my nursing shift early one morning, concentrating on a meeting that I was to have later that day, when suddenly, I found my regal car, Princess, I called her, kissing the side of a big new van. And we two were the only cars in the whole lot! Where was I? Certainly not in the moment, or else my Princess and I would have safely cleared the van.

The four principles of a spiritual warrior as taught by Confucius are: *Show up; pay attention; tell the truth from your heart, let go of the outcome.*

That day that Danu spoke her words to me, and *I got it,* I began to see the world through different eyes. All of a sudden I could see (not to mention feel the pain of) how ludicrous and inhumane it is to torture and maim a horse in order to produce a synthetic hormone for women when the humble soybean provides the same thing. I realized that organic food, besides tasting better, does not pump dangerous antibiotics and hormones into our bodies; I saw the good sense in recycling, and hugging trees no longer seemed so foolish. Now I feel blessed to be able to spread my energy of love to all whom I encounter.

Helen Paulus is founder of *Out of the Box Institute.* She studied with Deepak Chopra and became a Meditation and Yoga Instructor through the Chopra Center. She has attracted such people into her life as Wayne Dyer, Jack Canfield, Stephen Covey, Dennis Waitely, Marshall Rosenberg, Tony Robbins, Arielle and Debbie Ford, and Marianne Williamson. Helen has kindly offered to show how meditation uncovers the wonder and magic in the lives of others.

WANT BALANCE? MEDITATE

Just twenty minutes twice a day changed my world. The gift of meditation can change your world also.

Meditation leads to the magic of synchronicity. When asked what the single most important aspect of living the life I Love, the answer remains meditation. It led me to reveal my purpose statement:

"The purpose of my life is to wake up every day learning, growing, and attracting others also excited about learning and growing."

My purpose statement has evolved, yet the essence is part of my core.

Deepak Chopra in his book, *The Seven Spiritual Laws of Success,* says everyone born contains a unique talent and a special way of expressing that talent. To express *your* unique talent through "The Law of Dharma" (Purpose in Life), you want to make several commitments.

The first commitment: I am going to seek my higher self, which transcends my ego through spiritual practice. (Meditation);

The second commitment: I am going to discover my unique talents, and finding my unique talents, I am going to enjoy myself because the process of enjoyment occurs when I go into timeless awareness. That's when I am in the state of bliss. (Having fun);

The third commitment: I am going to ask myself how I am best suited to serve humanity. I am going to answer that question and put it into practice. I am going to use my unique talents to serve the needs of my fellow human beings; I will match those needs to my desire to help and serve others. (Do what I love to do).

Since I began meditating in 1997, I live a very synchronistic life. Like magic, thoughts and ideas to support my purpose unfold before me, and in the puzzle that is the bigger picture, my pieces fit. I meet the person for the job, find the building for the event and see money where I did not see it before. Magic happens all the time. Meditation allows us the stillness necessary to recognize the magical synchronicities all around us. Invite magic into *your* life with the following technique:

Mindfulness Meditation

1.   Close your eyes

2.   Gently allow your awareness to be on your breathing. Simply observe your breath as you breathe in and out.

3.   Just be aware of your breathing. Do not try to control or alter it in any way.

4. As you observe your breathing, you may notice that it changes in some way. It may get faster or slower, deeper or shallower. There may even be times when it appears to fade away completely. No matter how you're breathing changes, continue to observe it innocently, without resisting or changing it.

5. At times your attention will drift away from your breath to thoughts in your mind, sounds in the environment, or sensations in your body. Whenever you realize you are not observing your breath, gently bring your attention back to your breathing.

6. Remember to let go of any expectations you may have about the practice. If you notice that you are focusing on a mood or emotions, even looking for a particular experience, treat this like any other thought and bring your awareness back to your breathing. Let any thought or sensation pass like a cloud in the sky.

7. Now continue meditating gently for at least twenty to thirty minutes.

8. When time is up, keep your eyes closed, stop observing your breath and relax.

9. With your eyes closed, you can start to move and stretch your body, bringing your awareness back to the sounds and smells in the room.

10. When you are ready, and only when you feel ready, you can open your eyes.

You may choose to begin with an intention. When I first began meditation, I used a prayer from "A Course in Miracles" to set my intention. It goes like this:

I am responsible for what I see

I chose the feelings I experience

I set the goals I will achieve

Everything that seems to happen to me,

I asked for and receive as I have asked

And I ask for—List your request and then let them go like a helium balloon being released to the Universe.

Today I go into meditation with the *intention* of having anything that is in highest good of *all* flow through me with ease and grace.

Initially, I was unable to sit for more than five minutes; there was much more to do than sit still. I would do the dishes, clean the house, water flowers, anything to not be still. Little by little I increased the time, and now I can literally meditate for a few hours without interruption. Usually I practice thirty minutes twice a day. It is believed the best time is sunrise and sunset, when we are most connected to the rhythms of nature.

Start with whatever you are able to do, without judgment. Keep in mind there are many studies on the *proven benefits to health and wellness* meditation provides. In 1978, Robert Keith Wallace completed a ten-year study of meditators. He evaluated their biological age using three indicators: blood pressure, hearing, and near point vision. He found that the subjects who meditated for five years or less were on average five years younger biologically, and that subjects who had *meditated more than five years were on average twelve years younger biologically*, e. g. sixty-year olds had forty-eight-year old bodies. I know of physicians who recognize the power of meditation and place a sign on their office door that says "Do not disturb, Meditating."

Many of the people we admire and look up to meditate. They achieve a very strong sense of their purpose and live it. We are irresistibly attracted to them because of the light that shines through them. I believe living our purpose allows the world to give us exactly what we want. It is magnetized to us through our clear well defined intention and purpose.

Give yourself the *gift* of *meditation*, identify your purpose, your puzzle piece, and give others permission to do the same. The magic we experience ripples out every time we meditate. It is like throwing a pebble into the Universal pond.

Today, "The purpose of my life is to inspire others to embrace and express their light with fun, love and laughter."

Take Home Pearls

✧ We hear things only when we are ready to receive them.

✧ Meditation helps us live our purpose.

✧ Religion separates; spirituality unites.

✧ The magical practice of meditation invites synchronicities into your life.

✧ Meditators age 12 years later than non-meditators.

✧ Self love, taking our needs *first*, is key!

Chapter 17

Giving It All Away

Do you want to know how to stay healthy? Fill your heart with love—then give it away. Give it to all you meet, especially to those who have hurt you; to those whose beliefs are alien to you; to someone all alone and in despair. Perfect health is the sum of many parts, and the mind-body-spirit connection is what assures this.

As a well-known holistic physician, women, and sometimes men, flock from many states to see me, hoping I will fix their hormones and make them more balanced. The irony is that they come, assuming I have the answers. Yet, I shock them into the awareness that it is *they* who will fix them: I am merely a catalyst.

My mantra is the quote by the great physician, Albert Schweitzer: "The doctor is sent to entertain the patient while God does the healing." The simplicity and profundity in these words is often beyond our grasp: we think health is an elusive gift given only to the chosen few, when, in fact, is the birthright of all.

How you ask? Well, I am a menopause expert, trained as an herbalist, and in the use of bio-identical hormones. Three of my clinical research trials have been published in peer-reviewed journals. Yet, this aspect is such a small part of the picture. The greater, more vital aspect is what is going on in our souls.

We are, to be sure, spiritual beings having a human experience. Everything—I mean everything that manifests on our physical body — bubbles up from our soul. So, if my patient prostitutes herself to stay in a loveless marriage for its material comforts, she will never have perfect health. Her unhappiness will result in a multitude of physical ailments, from subtle to blatant, real to be sure, but having no distinct cause. And of course, conventional medicine comes to the rescue with band aid therapies for their pain: Motrin, Aleve, codeine, Vioxx (oh, sorry, this one was taken off the market after disclosure that major safety problems with this drug were hidden by an immoral scientist). But no one ever asks why they have the pain in the first place.

Let me tell you an amazing story. One of my teachers, Carolyn Myss, Ph.D., related it. She and her then partner, Norm Shealy, M.D., were conducting a workshop. There amongst the many attendees was a woman, lying on a cot, seemingly near death. It was said that she was riddled with cancer throughout her entire body. She had little time left to live. She did not stir, she did not speak, and she appeared as if in coma. The workshop was about forgiveness and the powerful healing that can come as a result of it.

The workshop ended, and to everyone's amazement, the woman in the so-called coma suddenly awoke, rose, and walked out into the night, never to be heard from again. Or so they thought....

Some five years later, Dr. Shealy arrived at an airport and was to be picked up by a driver and taken to a venue for a workshop. To his shock, the driver was none other than this woman.

"Do tell me your story," he implored.

She began:

"My husband had multiple affairs, starting on our

wedding day. Soon afterwards, my sons were born, and there was much to do, so leaving my husband was out of the question. Then, time passed, and the boys grew up and enlisted in the military service. They were sent to Vietnam. So surely I could not leave my husband then, for I worried day and night about my boys, and there was much work to be done. Finally, home safe from the war, my sons were reunited with us, and my worries about them over. All the stress and anger and resentment that I had stuffed these many years belched out of my soul and ravaged my body with cancer.

There seemed to be nothing left for me, and I prepared to die. Then I came to this powerful workshop, and listened with my heart to the words taught there. I then realized that despite all the hurt and abuse from my husband, I loved him. In that moment, I completely forgave him, and in that moment of forgiveness, I was healed."

Our stories are so vital, and yet we physicians are given fifteen minutes with each patient. (I see twenty-five patients every day.) I call upon my spirit guides and ask the Universe to conspire to slow down time, so that each patient can tell her story so that I may assist with the right therapy. If she has been sexually or physically abused in the past, and has never healed, my "treatment" is to implore them to counsel with a well-trained therapist who can bring this painful shadow into the light for healing. You may be shocked to know that in this world of 6.5 billion souls, two thirds have experienced abuse.

You ask—what does this have to do with love? Well, my friends, it has *everything* to do with it.

Why do we feel such a heart opening experience when we see a baby or a kitten or puppy? They are expressions of pure, unconditional love. They do not judge, they do not give you only part of their love. They give it all. That place where love and joy and peace and passion reside is the same place where hatred and resentment and non-forgiveness become a hard, dead stone. When the bard, Shakespeare, uttered the words, "Go to your bosom, knock there, and ask your heart what it doth know," he did not say "ask your *mind* what it doth know," he said, "heart." St. Francis of Assisi referred to the mind as Satan's lawyer. Even the Beatles knew that all you need is love.

I have made many observations over the years: even if a patient adheres to the basic tenets of good physical health, if she has "stinking thinking," she will never be healthy. By the same token, if our physical bodies are not healthy, our minds are sloppy and filled with lazy torpor.

Quantum physics, biblical teaching, Jesus and all the great teachers all agree: what we think, we become. That which we resist, persists. There are so many ways to say the same thing: we must focus on what it is that we desire, not on what we do not desire.

We all want and need love. You know of the classic observation: premature babies in an intensive care department thrived so dramatically when besides the physical comforts provided, they were held, loved, kissed. And we can only receive that healing love when we give it away. And as we are all sparks of the divine, giving love starts with me: *I must love me unconditionally and compassionately before I can receive it from others.*

HUGS HEAL

There is data to support that hugs heal. In fact, one hug gives much healing, two hugs give more, and somewhere around ten hugs daily give us an optimum dose of healing love. Actually, research states that we need four hugs to survive, eight for maintenance, and twelve for growth.

Let me tell you about Mary. She was a patient who came to see me. And my antennae were perched for hearing her story. As it is with many of my patients, she grew up in a very dysfunctional family. In fact, her father had sexually abused her from the time she was five years old. The abuse continued until she was eighteen years old, when she finally left home. Feeling lower than a pissant, entirely inconsequential, irrelevant and worthless, she drifted from relationship to relationship and job to job, never feeling good about herself and her ability. Her complaint during our visit together was painful sex, and chronic herpes infections.

Metaphysically, herpes represents shame and guilt. Mary had never counseled about her horrible abuse: in fact, I was the very first person to ever hear her story, and that was only because I *asked*.

Physicians know they need to ask about abuse, but many are either afraid of the answers or fearful that the story might take up too much time. If we do find out what is troubling our patients, often we don't know what to do about it. I have been blessed to be able to offer comfort, but more importantly, to guide these women into proper counseling. A magnificent Master's trained therapist, herself a victim of incest, helps my lovely women see that they did not cause the abuse, that they are whole and healed, that they simply need to first *forgive* themselves, most important, and then their abuser. I say *simply* because once we make a choice to do this, it happens spontaneously. This is the essence of self-esteem...and grace.

Each of my patients knows that at the end of their visit they can expect a hug from me, their doctor. I tell this story because Mary, unlike the thousands of patients I see every year, could not allow me to hug her. She would recoil and begin dressing. When I asked her why she could not be touched—although I knew the reason—she responded that each time someone embraced her, it brought her back to her abuse, the same reason she could not stay in a relationship that could be loving and nurturing. I could see that because she didn't feel worthy, she was sabotaging her happiness.

A happy sequel to this is that several months after Mary began her counseling, she came back to my office for a visit, and excitedly announced that she had found a partner and they would be getting engaged soon. And as she left, she gave me a long, grateful hug.

IN TO ME SEE

When each of you comes to see me as a patient, I offer you a trick question: "What are you doing good for yourself?" For you see, when you answer nothing, I realize that my job is more daunting than ever. If you are doing nothing good for yourself, how can you do good for anyone or anything else?

My teaching over and over is that we are mother martyrs, taking everyone else's needs first, and leaving ourselves on vapors. Do you realize what a dysfunctional and dangerous role model you are providing for your very impressionable children? Do you not see how you are creating another very unhealthy generation of mother martyrs? After the age of five, your children hear nothing that you say: they watch you, and when your actions contradict your words, the bullshit monitor begins ticking.

The deep grooves played into the record of self-derision and self-criticism need to be erased, and there is no other way to do this than to give yourself unconditional love. Not just when you are having a good hair day, or when you were particularly brilliant at the board meeting, or when you scored 220 at the bowling alley, but *always*. You have no trouble demonstrating unconditional love to a newborn baby, or to an adorable kitten or puppy, so why do you struggle showing yourself the same?

Of course, we struggle with self esteem: our being not enough has been imprinted on our very cellular matrix. Now it is time to stand, head held high in our self-love and utter the most important affirmation that we can muster: *I am a woman of power*!

HOW TO HEAL THE WORLD

One of the ways that I stay focused and in the now, which, by the way, is the only place that God is, is to utter "I love you" to each and every car that passes. By the time I arrive at work I am so immersed in love and compassion and patience that my day sails by.

Over sixty years ago, the father of quantum theory, Max Planck, shocked the world by stating that there is a "matrix" out there that provides the blueprint for the material world. More importantly, this place of pure energy is where are born the stars, our deepest relationships, peace in the world—first between individuals, then between peoples and nations, and even our DNA. The difference—and this is a powerful one—from the way we have been taught to look at this, is that our *beliefs* guide how our DNA will respond. The idea of our being victims of our genes is passé. The work of the modern-day biologist, Bruce Lipton, Ph.D., in *The Biology of Belief*, confirms this almost shocking concept.

Do we see how powerful we are? From the accepted dogma of our lives being outer directed, we see the power of being inner directed, through our heart-mind. Carl Jung says that he who looks outside, dreams; he who looks inside knows.

My patient, Irene, today a prominent lawyer, with four flourishing young adult children told me her story:

> *"I was born to my mother and a one-night stand whom I never knew. Having been the youngest of six children, I was shipped away to live with an aunt, herself burdened with five children, and finding me yet another. I was given many chores around the house, and at the age of eight, I cared for the three youngest after dragging home from school with barely three hours of sleep each night because the youngest had croup, and I had to stand in the hot shower with him to help his breathing.*
> *"This slavery lasted through high school, after which I ran*

away with a boyfriend who repeatedly raped and drugged me. He literally sold me into prostitution, and my need for the drugs, which seemed my only friends, got stronger and stronger. At twenty one, I ran away and signed myself into a rehab where, for the first time in my life, someone showed me kindness and an interest in what happened to me.

"I began working as a waitress, and taking night classes for college credits. I found my beloved. Strange, I was walking toward a table, deep in concentration as I totaled another customer's check, and when I looked up, I found myself immersed in the bluest, most loving eyes I had ever seen.

"George and I were married four months later, and he fostered my schooling fulltime. Two years later I was in law school, and found my dream to help runaways find their souls, as I had been privileged to do."

So many of us would have given up, yet the indomitable spirits that runs through us takes these challenges and turns them into precious opportunities to find our divine mission. I can't do yours, you can't do mine. Yet, the God-self of each of us has this mission to be the light of the world, and when my light and your light joins up, there is an exponential glow that joins up with other lights and then the magic begins.

Take Home Pearls

✧ Everything on our physical body bubbles up from our soul.

✧ Our very DNA can be changed with our beliefs.

✧ Research has found that we need four hugs to survive, eight for maintenance, and twelve to thrive.

✧ Adversity gives us the courage to strive for success.

✧ Self love, taking our needs *first*, is key!

Postscript

Things I've Learned in the Past Ten Years

Okay, dear readers, here is where I free associate all my thoughts, experiences, and Ahas. No rhyme or reason for the order of these things...

Yes, we pump antibiotics and hormones into animals to fatten them for the kill. These additives wreak havoc with our sacred bodies. It might be wise of us to learn the lesson of the Natives. They bless and honor with sacred cedar and extend their gratitude when they slay an animal, such as a deer, for food, so that the energy can be balanced. When we show continued gratitude for the animals that lay down their lives for us, the energy of reciprocity prevails. My treasured friend, Thalia, Greek Goddess and magnificent cook, reminds me never to mess about in the kitchen when angry, or sad, as those emotions taint the food and disturb our digestion.

Yes, we glamorize violence and continue fighting wars globally in the name of freedom and democracy; meanwhile thousands of people daily hold vigil in Assisi, Italy, honoring God and love.

Eating organically is important, especially if our animals are honored. But when eating out, simply bless the food and ask that it be fit for our sacred portals, our bodies.

Yes, we shake our fists at other drivers, get angry at workmates, and yell at spouses, but remember, we all are one. We possess aspects of everyone else, as well as what we consciously view as ourselves. Holy—wholistic—wholeness—all root forms for what we are.

Ah, my favorite subject: sex. Women cannot give themselves to lovemaking if they are seething in resentment at some real or imagined wrong perpetrated on us by, perhaps, our spouse. Communication is key: if we hold on to anger instead of gently—in non-accusatory fashion—discussing our feelings, we compound the hurt and misunderstanding. And since I am on the subject of sex: remember that after the age of forty our brain becomes our sex organ. Please reminisce back to the teens and twenties when our genital lust preceded everything we did. Other than getting good grades in school, there were few distractions.

What do we have now: jobs, mortgages, elderly parents, children, grandchildren, husbands with erectile dysfunction and stress, stress, stress! So, of course, a pillow is more inviting than a penis! The good news is that genital lust does not vanish, it just moves up to our brain, now the unadorned sex organ.

Ninety-nine percent of my patients admit that although they have no desire to initiate sex, once they get started, they love it. And so many of them muse why they do not dot it more often. So, my pretties, *make dates!* You do not arrive at a New York City play without reservations, right? Well, plan what you will wear, the music you will play, the sexy teddy you will sport. And play, play, play, using fruit in your belly buttons and invite each other to be a human fruit bowl.

All of this planning is a metaphor for waking up to our divinity: waking up to our feelings, to those emotions that crash and burn us, because we react to every word and behavior of another with a defensiveness and righteousness as if we are perfect beings.

Please let me remind you that we co-create every aspect of our lives, not consciously, most often, because we would be horrified to hear so starkly that the many dramas in life are brought on by our thoughts, words, and behaviors.

Did I really say that? Did I dare suggest that the sexual and physical abuse at the hand of your father was in some part invited by you? Did I dare suggest that you orchestrated the birth of your bipolar children and your embezzler husband? Did I willfully marry three men that would ultimately abuse me physically and emotionally, driving me to suicide?

The answer is best shown by the understanding that we are spiritual beings having a human experience and not the other way around. We are, to be sure, as Teillard de Chardin says, collaborators in creation. That God, thought to be up there, so separate and distinct from us, is in fact, within us. These experiences, some horrifying to be sure, are but lessons to bring us closer to our divinity. These are not punishments, but precious gifts that constantly bring us closer and closer to that unconditional love and compassion which is our true birthright.

The question I asked, all these long years from the age of sixteen with my first boyfriend, Freddie, (the chocolate chip cookie boy, remember?) until nigh on my sixty-fifth year on planet earth was: "How can I change to make you love me more?" The question should have been "How can I love *me* more?" because "I am enough just the way I am."

We are mirrors for each other, and we create our very experiences over and over and over until we learn the lesson we were sent here to learn.

We are powerful enough to create our reality with consciousness, and yes, enlightenment—a term the Buddha uses to remind us that we are awake.

So the journey continues; the onion peels, and each and every day, I am respectful of my need to remain vigilant so as to never go back to that place of fear and not-enoughness.

Epilogue

Recently, after four years of being alone and working mightily to heal the wounds of my eventful, dramatic past, I made a list of what I wanted in my life's partner:

- He will have grey hair
- He will love to dance
- He will love cats
- He will be healthy, sexy, and playful
- He will be abundant
- He will have been on his spiritual journey

And God, I know I am asking a lot, but can he have an apartment in New York City?

In 2007 four psychics told me that I would meet my beloved in August of that year. Flying to Greece for my best friend's daughter's wedding, I arrived with one of the four the night before the wedding, which was to be celebrated September 1. We arrive after a long, convoluted trip through France, finding DeGaul Airport a daunting and confusing place. Of course, we missed our connection to Aegina, the magnificent island hosting the wedding. Finally, sleepy, weary travelers, upon arriving, we nonetheless chose to sit in an outdoor café, reveling in anticipation of the festivities that next day.

"Rose, I said: "Do your realize that it is quarter to eleven? The bewitching hour, according to you?

You psychics know nothing. I am going to turn into a pumpkin. I am not going to meet my beloved!"

Then it happened: that Kismet time when our life's journey falls into our laps, and we gasp—it is so.

Jakob walked by with his cousin, Sura. We met and the prophecy was fulfilled.

I liked his face immediately, and cheekily asked of Sura, "Who is your date?"

"This is not my date" she responded: "This is my cousin, Jack."

She reminded me later that a smile of relief crossed my face, as if I remembered the prediction in its fullest meaning.

Jack and I sat together at the reception that following day, chattering like magpies, each wanting to know more and more about each other. He was sixty, I sixty five when we met. He is an only child; I am an only child. I have a single child, my son Basil. He has a single child, his daughter Erin. I have had three divorces, he has had one. That evening, we closed down two discos following the reception. Finally at five in the morning, I acknowledged fatigue, but we vowed to meet on the beach the following day.

So here I go again, I thought. But I also thought, *this is different.* Two earth-spinning stops jolted my awareness: I remembered my list of "conditions" put to paper eight months prior: grey hair, cats, dance, healthy, sexy, playful, abundant, spiritual. Would he have an apartment in New York?

Well, my sisters, be careful what you ask for, because you just might get it. I got it all, including the apartment in New York City, on

Sutton Place, owned by Sura and generously on loan when we are in New York City. This all sound so schmaltzy, but the more important occurrence took place three months before that fateful day. I awoke that day, looked in the mirror, and said, "Helene, you are *enough*. You no longer have to change to make someone love you: it is *you* you need to love."

Jakob is the mirror into which I gaze each morning: as I love myself, I am capable of loving this magnificent man who loves to play squash, loves the New York Yankees, loves cats, loves to dance, and loves Heineken beer. And of course he loves me, just as I am.

We do not have agendas, we have work to do on our respective souls: that includes acknowledging that ego (edging God out) will find occasion to rise, and perhaps cause some mayhem around issues such as breathing space, power, viewpoints, living conditions, jobs or travel. But those are issues representing the dualism created by the illusion of this physical world.

I find that our love and connection more resembles that teaching by the God of all that is: love unconditionally, forgive unconditionally—first yourself then the other. Serve and fill the cup, first of self then of other. Create peace, first in your heart, then in the other.

As long as I keep the pretense of being human, I must remain vigilant over my forty year journey of self loathing. I need to ever forgive my flaws, my foolishness, my arrogance, remembering that as a spiritual being having a human experience I am given this opportunity to express my divinity, my perfect self love.

It is time in the evolution of the feminine that we no longer play small. Though we just received the vote only less than a century ago, though we still walk ten paces behind in some cultures, and still women are being deprived of their clitoris in male-dominated areas to deprive us women of our sexual joy—nonetheless, it is time that the masculine and feminine energies merge to bring forward on our tattered planet a new energy that recognizes love as our fuel and compassion as the way to that love.

RESOURCES

ALLIANCE FOR A NEW HUMANITY
400 Calle Calaf PMB 460 Suite 233
San Juan, Puerto Rico 00918
newsletter@anhglobal.org
www.anhglobal.org

Started by Deepak Chopra and Arsenio Rodriguez, its mission is to connect people who, through personal and social transformation, aim to build a just, peaceful, and sustainable world reflecting the unity of all humanity.

AMERICAN HOLISTIC MEDICAL ASSOCIATION
23366 Commerce Park Suite 101B
Beachwood, Ohio 44122
216-292-6644
info@holisticmedicine.org
www.holisticmedicine.org

Started thirty-one years ago by visionaries such as Gladys McGarey, M.D., Norm Shealy, M.D., this dedicated group of holistic and integrative physicians are a beacon for the way medicine can be when we combine the best of science with the heart of medicine.

APOLLO NUTRITION
3556 Apollo Court
Orefield, PA 18069-2601
877-527-6556 (5 APOLLO)

Tom Maslar, my friend and fellow herbalist, blends a great assortment of only the highest quality herbs and nutrients into a green powder known as Nature's Greens, and is the main addition to my very healthy nutritional shake that starts my day.

CAROLYN DEAN, M.D., N.D., resides in Maui. She has authored and coauthored seventeen health books, has a complimentary online newsletter, online health courses, and a busy telephone consulting practice. You will enjoy what Dr. Dean has to offer at www.drcarolyndean.com.

DR. DAVID WILLIAMS
Mountain Home Nutritionals
700 Indian Springs Drive
Lancaster, PA 17601
www.drdavidwilliams.com

Dr. Williams, a chiropractor by training, has traveled worldwide to locate, evaluate, formulate and write about proven treatments and cures for practically every major health concern today.

DR. RICHARD SCHULTZE
American Botanical Pharmacy
4114 Glencoe Avenue
Marina Del Rey, CA 90292
1-800-herb-doc
www.herbdoc.com

Dr. Schultze, master herbalist, teaches us how to achieve and maintain vibrant health, especially through colon cleansing and eating only pure organic food. He adds garlic to many of his herbal preparations, which greatly enhances their potency.

EMERITA
1339 NE Airport Way Suite 200
Portland OR 97230
503-226-1010 or 1-800-648-8211 tele.
503-226-6455 or 1-800-944-0168 fax
Customer service 1-800-888-6041
www.emerita.com

This woman-owned company started as a family business in the 1970s. Sharon MacFarland, CEO, features natural wellness products, the best known of which is Pro-Gest, natural transdermal progesterone cream, a major component of my bioidentical hormone regimens.

GLADYS TAYLOR MCGAREY MEDICAL FOUNDATION
4848 E. Cactus Road Suite 505-506
Scottsdale, AZ 85254
480-946-4544 tele.

The foundation, begun by Gladys McGarey, M.D., promotes and provides education, research, and development that guide individuals and communities to engage in their own healing, creating living medicine in a living environment.

HERBALIST & ALCHEMIST
51 South Wandling Avenue
Washington, NJ 07882
908-689-9020 tele.
908-689-9071 fax
www.herbalist-alchemist.com

This excellent company is run by David Winston, an internationally known lecturer, author, and ethnobotanist for more than thirty-five years.

NATURAL RESOURCES DEFENSE COUNCIL
40 West 20th Street
New York, New York 10011
212-727-4500 tele.
212-727-1773 fax
www.nrdc.org

Out of every dollar contributed to this worthy organization, seventy-nine cents goes directly to NRDC Environmental Programs, helping save our precious natural resources.

NATIONAL SPEAKERS ASSOCIATION
1500 South Priest Drive
Tempe, AZ 85281
480-968-2552 tele.
480-968-0911 fax
www.nsaspeaker.org

This magnificent organization gave me courage to step out as a professional speaker by teaching me the science of public speaking. My colleagues are always ready and willing to assist my becoming better and better as I develop the art and science of sharing my wisdom.

ORGANIC CONSUMERS ASSOCIATION
6771 South Silver Hill Drive
Finland, MN 55603
218-226-4164 tele.
218-353-7652 fax
www.organicconsumers.org

OCA is an online and grassroots nonprofit [501(c) 3] public interest organization campaigning for health, justice, and sustainability.

OUT OF THE BOX INSTITUTE
610-770-9972 tele.
610-740-0638 fax
www.outoftheboxinstitute.com

Helen Paulus, mentor, certified meditation and yoga instructor through the Chopra Center and affectionately known as "The Out of The Box Mentor-For Life" fulfills her life purpose by empowering others to search for and find their purpose. She facilitates a highly-successful teleconference program steeped in the wisdom of her mentor, Deepak Chopra and his book, "The Seven Spiritual Laws of Success" The "Zero to Abundance in 77 Days" program provides magical, yet practical tools to reveal purpose, abundance, and balance in all aspects of life.

SHERRILL SELLMAN, N.D.
WomanWise International
450 W. 7th St Suite 1502
Tulsa, OK 74119
Tel: 918-728-7068 Cell: 918-720-4865
golight@earthlink.net
http://www.whatwomenmustknow.com

Sherrill Sellman, N.D., is an internationally acclaimed holistic women's health advocate. She is the best-selling author of *Hormone Heresy: What Women MUST Know* and *What Women MUST Know to Protect Their Daughters fro Breast Cancer*. She is the host of a national radio show, *What Women MUST Know* at www.prncomm.net. Dr. Sellman consults with women via phone consultations. She can be contacted at golight@earthlink.net or call 918-728-7069. Her educational website www.whatwomenmustknow.com offers many free articles and audio lectures.

SHERRY ROGERS, M.D.
Prestige Publishing
PO Box 3068
Syracuse, NY 13220
1-800-846-6687
www.prestigepublishing.com

Dr. Rogers has authored thirteen books on original scientific material and lectures worldwide. She is a foremost authority on Allergy, Immunology, and Environmental Medicine, and I have been enlightened by her newsletter and books for the past eighteen years.

THE NATURE CONSERVANCY
4245 N Fairfax Drive   Suite 100
Arlington, VA 22203
1-800-628-6860
nature.org

This important organization is always on the front line, ready to protect another landscape or waterscape where they put their science-based expertise to work. They work hard to protect nature for future generations.

THE WESTON A. PRICE FOUNDATION
PMB #106380
4200 Wisconsin Avenue NW
Washington, DC 20016
202-363-4394 tele.
202-363-4396 fax
www.westonaprice.org

The Weston A. Price Foundation is a non-profit, tax-exempt charity founded in 1999 to disseminate the research of nutrition pioneer, Dr. Weston Price, whose studies of isolated nonindustrialized peoples established the parameters of human health and determined the optimum characteristics of human diets: they must consist of nutrient-dense, whole foods and the vital fat-soluble activators found exclusively in animal fats.

WOMEN'S WISDOM AND WELLNESS
610-776-7045
www.womenswisdomwellness.com

Tahya and Dr. Helene Leonetti present Women's Wisdom & Wellness, an interactive program designed to reveal truths of well-being.

Dr. Helene provides insights into realizing your Self-Esteem Gene, and the Tahya Technique activates it, rekindling each woman's unique spark of femininity, love, and creativity. Together they facilitate a mind/body/spirit journey toward an elegant, elevated sense of self. This program is suitable for women of all ages, all shapes and sizes. Tapping into our Self-Esteem Gene is vital for our evolution.

VIRGINIA HOPKINS HEALTH WATCH
www.virginiahopkinstestkits.com

Virginia Hopkins brings science to alternative medicine and common sense to conventional medicine. She co-authored two best-selling books with Dr. John Lee, including the classic, "What Your Doctor May Not Tell You About Menopause," and writes the Virginia Hopkins Health Watch, an e-mail newsletter about natural hormones for women and men, nutrition news, prescription alternatives, and much more!

ZRT LABORATORY
8605 SW Creekside Place
Beaverton, OR 97008
503-466-2445 tele.
503-466-1636 fax
www.zrtlab.com

David Zava, Ph.D., has been testing hormone levels in saliva and blood spot sampling, and is intimately involved in transdermal progesterone research. He coauthored the excellent book with John R. Lee, MD, "What Your Doctor May Not Tell You About Breast Cancer."

Nurturing Yourself to Vibrant Health

Helene Leonetti, M.D., has experienced her own personal trauma, yet now lives and works in a state of healthy peace, acceptance, and gratitude. That transformation is the core of *Hardwired for Love*. Her story, and the teaching of wisdom gained through her journey, reflects a guided path to wholeness and health that all women can take to heart.

Far too many women are living with a desperate combination of unhealthy bodies, psychological issues, and spiritual deadness. In Dr. Leonetti's new book you'll discover:

- How your thoughts create your reality and what you can do to clarify your thinking
- Why you're safer on a bridge between conventional medicine and holistic healing
- Healthy solutions to chronic pain, menopause, digestive, psychological, and sexual issues
- The freedom of unconditional love, compassion and forgiveness toward yourself

"Dr. Leonetti is every woman's dream gynecologist . . . respectful, compassionate, competent in both traditional and complementary medical approaches, honest , and very human. Her book shares wisdom gained over her personal and professional lifetime. She is an inspiration to her patients, colleagues, and friends."

—Sherrill Sellman, N.D.
author of *What Women MUST Know* book series
Senior Editor, Total Health Magazine

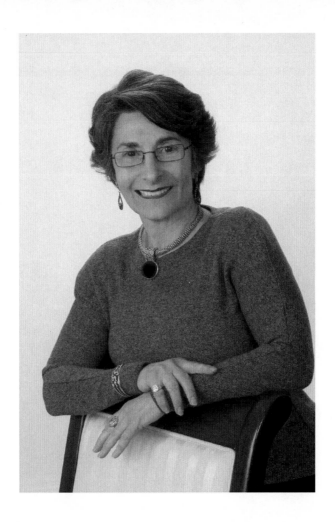

Helene Leonetti, M.D., is a board-certified OB-GYN physician and self-described "Gynechiatrist," with a thriving practice in Bethlehem, Pennsylvania. Her previous books include *Menopause: A Spiritual Renaissance*, and she is a contributor to *A Healthier You*, *Living In Clarity*, part of the highly popular *Wake Up...Live the Life You Love* series, and *Inspiring Hope*. Her practice is focused on joining the best of conventional medicine and holistic treatment, while awakening all women to the healing power of self-love and acceptance.

For more information and support, visit:
www.HardwiredForLove.com